Sandra,
Your support + ... is c... Tru... Cha...

ON HER PLATE

ON HER PLATE:
Plant-based recipes, life stories, and natural health sciences to align mind, body, and earth.
2018 Golden Brick Road Publishing House Inc.
Trade Paperback Edition
Copyright @ 2018 Ky-Lee Hanson

Published in Canada, Printed in China for Global Distribution by Golden Brick Road Publishing House Inc.
www.goldenbrickroad.pub

For more information email: kylee@gbrph.ca
ISBN: trade paperback 978-1-988736-41-9
ebook 978-1-988736-42-6
Mobi 978-1-988736-43-3

To order additional copies of this book: orders@gbrph.ca

The Women's Wellness Warriors present:

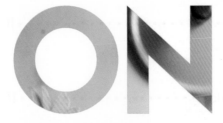

ON

Plant-based recipes, life stories,

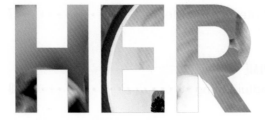

HER

and natural health sciences

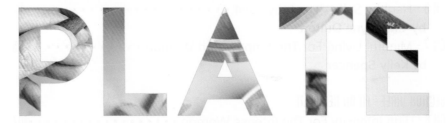

PLATE

to align mind, body, and earth.

KY-LEE HANSON

Tania Moraes-Vaz | Effie Mitskopoulos | Samantha Cifelli
Jenna Knight | Margie Cook | Paula Man | Kelly Spencer
Deirdre Slattery | Charleyne Oulton | Sindy Ng
Jy Nanda | Neli Tavares Hession | Allison Marschean
Rebecca Hall | Amy Rempel | Meghan Rose
The Plantiful Chef | Ashly Hill

CONTENTS

Be like a pineapple

STAND TALL,

WEAR A CROWN,

AND BE SWEET

ON THE INSIDE

Preface

by Ky-Lee Hanson

T he Women's Wellness Warriors are here to guide you through your day to day struggles, lift you up when you fall, and help you lead a more nourishing life. We are each here to share our pain, passion, and life lessons in order to band together with other women and take our world towards a brighter, more nurturing future. This book is not meant to tell you there is only *one* way to live, nor are we attempting to show you a perfect life or portray ourselves as being perfect. And we are certainly not here to preach or tell you what you are doing is wrong. We are here to embrace the perfectly imperfect and share real stories of how many women live, while offering to you, food for thought. Some of the biggest realizations I had about my own struggles and ailments came from hearing the honest stories of other women and listening to *what* they did to make their lives a little bit better. Their tips may not always work for me, but the sheer practice of sharing their truth and experiences, and their quest for holistic solutions as an option being presented, is the fuel I need, the REMINDER I need, to go out and explore what works best for *my* mind, body, and soul. I love to learn and practice the art of well-being, but I also seem to equally "love" overdoing it and getting into "busy" states of mind. A few years ago, I wrote a book titled *Dear Stress, I'm Breaking Up With You*, because I personally needed it and was sick and tired of people using that word passively. "Oh it's just stress," and "I am too busy." This is not an acceptable way to live. Before writing that book, I was on a journey to rid expectations, to gain confidence, and to become more level in my communications with others. I achieved all this. I achieved career success too, and along the way found "purpose." Purpose to live in a way that inspires others, a purpose to learn and share knowledge, a purpose to impact this world in a positive way. I realized I had influence. I realized all people do, but it is our choice to harness it or not. I chose the prior. A purpose is simply something that keeps you going. It's that simple - something that brings joy, change, healing, and innovative ideas to the world. It is not hard to do and be good, even just small things. We have little time here on earth and I decided to live in a positive, stress free, and impactful way.

Great! I did break up with stress, and my life is seriously a lot more calm. *I used to be a crazy person.* However, my body didn't come out completely on top. I learned to convey my message and energy into structured, positive execution, which also meant learning to control and calm myself when my blood wants to boil or when someone is driving me nuts. Now, I am the polar opposite on a calm-crazy spectrum compared to where I was three, five, and ten years ago. However, I did find myself becoming a stress eater. *Gasp!* *Did I just admit that and take responsibility, in writing?!* Taking responsibility is the strongest step towards self-awareness and points us towards the direction of healing and growth. I have always loved food, and luckily I love plant-based foods.

However, I did find myself becoming a stress eater.

Chips are "technically" a vegetable - *does that count?* And pizza, bread, crackers, pasta - *yum, simple carbohydrates!* Cheese or no cheese, just give me the grains! But seriously, I also love mangos, quinoa, broccoli, falafels, beans, vegan protein bars, *vegan anything really,* and nutrient shakes. These are my jam but not always the first tune I want to dance to. I have been gravitating towards the quick spikes, quick energy, quick jolts of pleasure, and eating for stimulation. *Since when do I like sugar?* I have eaten more chocolate and cake in these last two years than probably my entire life - *what is up with that?!* And I am certain, I am not the only person feeling this way. I am also not the only educated-in-health person who screws up on her diet. Although, I thought my break-up with stress was complete, in some ways, it just manifested in other areas. What I forgot was a holistic approach, the elusive "balanced" way of life. These things take time, they take further lessons, and they take more than one approach. We have to look at ourselves as a whole, yet acknowledge all the working parts. Firstly, mindset is important, and I had to start there to understand what is going on with me now - in my body.

So, I put an idea out there, and coauthors and readers jumped on it. I have a good sense for what is needed and when it is needed, and that is how this book came about: born from the awareness of both my needs and the needs of others by asking people what they struggle with. My hope is that you will gain some clarity into your own lifestyle through reading this book, *instead of having to write your own before figuring it out...* However, we do know that communication is the key to a healthy relationship as writing is a form of communication with the self. I encourage writing as my career; it brings about the answers that lie within. We discover the answers within us by searching, and we search through questioning.

You can learn more about my personal story, background, and education in my chapter. This book is filled with wellness warriors who share awesome tips they use with their clients, but to keep this from being an educational over-our-head snore, I helped them convey WHY they do what they do and what ailments they have or had, in order to help you see that even the educated struggle. You are no less of a woman for overeating, stressing, missing a workout, or feeling like you hate working out. You are probably MORE of a woman for these things! The point is, there is no perfect. There are things that commonly work and we will share those with you, but the main message of this book is...

Live in a way that makes YOU feel your best deep down. Collect information from *many* sources and many doctors, practice integrative medicine, which means to use many modalities, and decide for yourself what your body needs. The best thing I ever did and what helped me avoid organ removal, was getting a second opinion followed by my own research. Actually to be honest, I got five more opinions. I knew what I wanted to hear and I searched until I heard it. Listen to your body and work WITH your body. It knows best on what you need. Your body constantly tries to communicate with you, and we are going to help you listen to it.

with you, but the truth message of this book is....

Live in a way that makes YOU feel your best deep down. Collect information from many sources and many doctors, practice integrative medicine, which means to use many modalities, and decide for yourself what your body needs. The best things I ever did and what helped me avoid organ removal was getting a second opinion followed by my own research. Actually to be honest, I got five more opinions. I knew what I wanted to hear and I searched until I heard it. Listen to your body and work WITH your body. It knows best on what you need. Your body constantly tries to communicate with you, and we are going to help you listen to it.

Introduction

by Ky-Lee Hanson

O*n Her Plate*, explores the female interaction with society, the earth, both good and bad, chemicals in food and skincare, lifestyle factors affecting the human epigenome, the state of our environment, and women's health, fitness, and recipes. We are called The Women's Wellness Warriors because we are women focusing on our wellness against obstacles of society so we can then help other women. We rise for women, together as women. We aim to share knowledge and ideas to empower women as they are typically natural nurturers who love, care, and share; we are the best vehicle for birthing change. Men and children have the same macronutrient (proteins, fats, carbohydrates as well as dietary fiber and fluids) and micronutrient (vitamins and minerals) needs as women, but in different amounts. There are illnesses specifically known as *female* cancers and *female* hormonal conditions, as well as a lot more *generally* goes on in a woman, not only on a monthly basis, but also through labor and menopause. Our bodies live, react, and age differently than men. We deserve our own book. That is what this book will address. We will also share with you easy and affordable ways to be more earth friendly while nurturing your own health and the health of your family. Of course, much of our shared knowledge is also applicable to your family. We are cautious about human influence on our earth and how it affects the health of all beings on a global scale. When it comes to genetically modified organisms (GMOs) and pesticides, we look at long term effects, and its presence in a large variety of things we consume causing cumulative damage to our body and the earth. While society may find there are quantity, cost, and waste control benefits to feeding a growing, financially-distraught population, the actuality is, nature is nature. We are natural beings, and the earth has a natural rhythm. These chemicals disrupt that. As a society, we are wasteful in many ways and do not empower. Instead, we sometimes restrict cities and subdivisions around growing food and gardens. There are many other ways we can correct the world's problems. Even if GMOs are safe for consumption, the reality is, if these crops are not in a controlled environment, they cross pollinate and have effects on the environment and alter other strains of crops, the wild, land, and animals in adverse ways. Farmaid.org lists five top concerns about GMOs from a financial perspective and includes multiple cases and lawsuits - further proof that GMOs damage crops and land, and harm people. Many plants are pollinated by insects, birds or wind, allowing pollen from a GMO plant to move to neighboring fields or into the wild. This "genetic drift" illustrates the enormous difficulty in containing GMO Technology. "Not only is genetic drift impossible to prevent, inadequate regulation also fails to hold seed companies accountable..." In 2000, StarLink Com's corn–not approved for human consumption–is found in 300 food products. This article contains lawsuits up until 2014. GMOinside.org is another resource to learn about cross contamination. Jennifer Hsaio wrote a study for Harvard, GMOs and Pesticides: Helpful or Harmful? which stated, "According to the Natural Institute of Health, the health effects of pesticides are still not well understood... GMOs are often engineered to be resilient to pesticides or produce pesticides themselves." The questions, studies, experiences, and education from our authors explore what happens when we influences our earth's environment and our internal body environment in positive, negative, as well as unknown ways.

Your body is the coolest machine, and it is trying to work with you. As much as you may think it is failing you or that you are inadequate, or maybe you feel as though you are failing your body, this is simply not the case. There are simply obstacles that need to be dealt with, and we are here for that reason. Be conscious of your environment and the choices you make, and you will start to feel this new sense of communication and understanding with yourself. You will feel a new sense of calm and begin to live in a different light. You will start identifying triggers to the physical body instead of just triggers to the mind. The body feels its own triggers and stressors which we aren't always conscious of, but we can learn to be so from many authors in this book.

The amazing thing about a co-author book is, you are going to learn and experience shifts through many voices - some more serious, some more technical, and some more moving. Collectively, we want people to feel good; we want a healthy earth full of healthy bodies. We have come to realize that some people might just not know what healthy feels like anymore as we live in a society that promotes illness. First, we start you off with technical stuff, to help you understand the body, science, and how food is produced, followed by mindfulness and the mind / body connection. We then go into rich stories on specific conditions that are common to many women, with solutions and success stories. We focus both on physical body conditioning and internal hormonal balancing. Lastly, we give you food! We developed quick and familiar, nutrient packed meals to help you add more goodness into your week, easily. Health does not have to be complicated, and plant-based meals can be satisfying. This book focuses on the Divine connection we share with the earth. Women are typically natural nurturers, and our bodies, earth, and people of the world need us. We focus on plant-based, wholesome foods as a key in women's wellness. Plant-based means to have 80-100% of your plate consisting of foods from plants: herbs, vegetables, fruits, nuts, seeds, and grains. The most common diet labels to achieve this are: vegan, vegetarian (adding eggs and / or dairy), and pescatarian (including fish). Some less commonly referred to as "plant-based" but depending on each person's unique preferences, the following could fall within the 80/20 rule: paleo, flexitarian, and Mediterranean.

Plant-based nutrition is good disease prevention for women because heart disease is the leading cause of premature death amongst women. For example, the added fat in beef is saturated which may not be healthy if one is at risk for heart disease. Furthermore, the added fat elevates the calorie content without increasing the beneficial nutrients, which could hinder weight-loss or maintenance efforts if it causes you to eat too much for your activity level. Weight-gain can lead to a sea of other ailments and conditions such as osteoporosis. According to researchers at the Harvard School of Public Health, the added salt and preservatives found in processed cuts of red meat, such as bacon, sausage, and deli meats may increase cardiovascular disease risk. [1] And for the men in your life, in 2016, the International Agency for Research on Cancer from the World Health Organization (WHO) confirmed, "Consumption of processed meat was classified as carcinogenic and red meat as probably carcinogenic after the IARC Working Group – comprised of 22 scientists from ten countries – evaluated over 800 studies. Conclusions were primarily based on the evidence for colorectal cancer. Data also showed positive associations between processed meat consumption and stomach cancer, and between red meat consumption and pancreatic and prostate cancer."

"Veganism is a very fine form of nutrition. It's a little extreme to tell a person who is using flesh foods that you're going to take everything entirely away from them. When I was in practice in medicine, I would tell the patients that the vegetable-based diet was the healthy way to go, and to keep away from the animal products as much as possible. People are very sensitive about what they eat. You can talk to people about exercising, relaxation, good mental attitude and they will accept that. But you talk to them about what they are eating and people are very sensitive about that. If an individual is willing to listen, I will try to explain to them on a scientific basis of how I think it's better for them."

~ DR. ELLSWORTH WAREHAM

While there is much debate around the nutrients of meat, we are not here to discuss what is right or what is wrong; we are simply speaking on plants, cellular health, women's hormonal complications, the Divine connection to Mother Earth, and how as influential women, we must nurture and protect the environment. However, I came to learn the most nutrient dense meats are foods that most people do not frequently eat: liver, shellfish, and oysters. [2] As a plant-based person and while vegan for part of my life, I did always wonder why scallops were not a vegan food... this is a common gray area in the community as many discuss scallops and also mussels, act and feel pain in the same way a plant does, which created a new "label" called "Seagan": sea + vegan. *Seriously, look it up.* My point being, you don't need a label in order to do what feels right for your body.

Let's get started! To learn more from the sources we have studied, please see the references for citations at the back of the book and the glossary of terms. In addition, each chapter has a biography for the author of that chapter. We encourage you to reach out to these authors; *that is why their contact information is there!* Join our sisterhood, learn, and be surrounded by positivity so you can feel better. We also encourage you to research into the schools we have attended and sign up for some courses! Enjoy!

UNEARTH HER PLATE

Featuring

Rebecca Hall

Meghan Rose

Ky-Lee Hanson

FINDING BALANCE IN TODAY'S WORLD

DESIRE THAT WHICH YOU SEEK AND THE UNIVERSE WILL CONSPIRE TO MAKE IT REALITY.

by Rebecca Hall

Massage Therapist, MT | Yoga Teacher, YTT

Rebecca Hall

Rebecca was born on November 15th, 1978 in the beautiful state of Western Australia; a pristine region of forest, world class surf, jewel caves, home gardens, and rainwater catchment.

Rebecca has a fun and loving outlook on life. She loves to play and surf with friends, her six-year-old son, Levi, and sweet husband, Aaron. From a lifetime of self-transformation, Rebecca has a deep passion for the well-being of others and the planet.

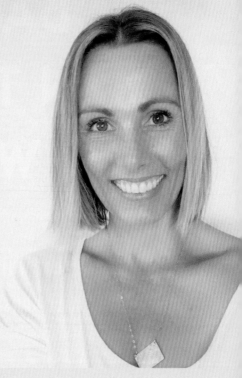

Rebecca has grown a highly successful private practice in massage therapy, yoga, and nutrition and has worked within her community for decades with some the most famous names in the world as her long term clients.

Rebecca is also a top leader and wellness coach for Purium Health Products - an organic non-GMO superfoods company, which has been recognized on the INC 5000 list for four consecutive years one of the fastest growing companies.

Rebecca has grown a fun loving organization of thousands that have gratefully brought balance into their health and lives. With some of the nation's top healthcare professionals and naturopathic doctors on her team, they continue to nourish others as they have nourished themselves into balance again.

WWW.KAUAIMASSAGEYOGAANDNUTRITION.COM
ig: rebeccahallkauai | Kauai massage yoga & nutrition
fb: Rebecca Hall | Kauai Massage, Yoga & Nutrition

Turning Back The Clock

I was extremely blessed to be born to my beautiful parents, Evelyn and Simon, and to grow up with my awesome brother, Chris. As a toddler, it was clear that I had physical imbalances in my body; my hips were rotated, my knees touched, and my feet crossed, causing me to trip whenever I walked.

At the young age of two, my mum began to seek corrective help for me through therapy, movement, and strengthening classes. By age fourteen, although I was playing high level sports despite my body form, I experienced chronic pain and inflammation. This is when my dad introduced me to his yoga teacher and yoga classes.

By age nineteen, I had my first knee surgery, was diagnosed by my orthopedic surgeon with severe arthritis in my knees and hips, and was told that I may need replacements as I grew older. Though my pain and inflammation was chronic, even unbearable at times, it didn't stop me.

When we moved to the island of Kauai in 2005, I incorporated structural integration therapy, plant-based medicine, education, food sourcing, and internal cleansing into my healing journey. We grew our own organic garden including medicinal plants like turmeric root, which is known for its healing and anti-inflammatory properties.

Despite all these holistic practices, my pain and inflammation was still there. My husband, Aaron, was also suffering with various ailments and had been for years. However, we didn't heal ourselves until we deeply nourished and cleansed our bodies through living superfoods.

Within five days, my arthritis pain and inflammation subsided and have shown no signs of returning for two years now.

Within seven days, Aaron's severe depression lifted, his pain and inflammation both gone, and we both sleep really well with no more chronic fatigue.

Educating ourselves deeply and being the change we wish to see is not only the greatest gift we can offer in service to ourselves and our families, but it can dramatically change the world, too.

Plant-based superfoods are plants, grains, legumes which have a dense nutritional value. They contain naturally occurring vitamins and minerals from the plant which are bioavailable to the body. There are everyday plant-based superfoods that can be consumed on a regular basis and also concentrated superfoods that can be consumed but in a smaller amount, offering the magic of bioavailable nutrients to our body and mind.

"Bioavailability" is the ease with which any nutrient can make its way from the food you eat into your body. The bioavailability journey that every nutrient takes is the same. In the first part of the journey, the food must be digested (broken apart) so that the nutrient can be free from the food that contained it. The second part of the journey involves absorption of the nutrient from the digestive tract into the rest of the body. Superfoods have a very high nutrient bioavailability. They can be digested and absorbed at a higher percentage of the time and in a dependable way.

Sadly, with the food crisis of today, the foods that are available have an extremely low bioavailability and little to zero nutrient value. The digestion and absorption of these foods can be much more difficult and less value to our body and mind, causing damage and inflammation to the gastrointestinal tract making it hard to assimilate nutrients properly, especially as most have binders, fillers, synthetics, chemicals, added hormones, and are genetically modified.

Educating ourselves deeply on where, who, and how our food source is coming to us can be the beginning of a complete transformation for yourself and your family. When we can deeply nourish our bodies with pure unadulterated foods, we can have enough energy and clarity to serve our community as well.

Full Circle

It's a Saturday morning here in Hawaii. I'm the first one awake and can hear the roosters crowing in the distance, I feel well rested and my body feels light. Though this was not the case for more than two decades, thankfully, it is now.

I make myself a green drink and move out onto the deck. I can feel the perfect temperature on my skin and smell the scent of tropical flowers being carried by on the Hawaiian breeze. As I look out to the mountains and reflect on this week's consultations, my mind has mixed emotions. Everyday I'm blessed to receive stories from family, friends, and clients about how their bodies, minds, and lives have positively changed for the better.

However, there are still so many new people I'm consulting with that are exhausted, stressed out, in debt, in pain, not sleeping, overweight, or underweight. There are so many more people with diabetes, autoimmune conditions, cancer, and other terminal illnesses, or facing death before the age of fifty. It's completely heartbreaking. Why are we seeing more and more people suffering? What has changed with our world today?

A Bigger Perspective

If we were astronauts and looked at the view of our planet from space, it would be a life changing experience and a massive "agent of change" once we got back down to the ground on earth.

Well this is exactly how Ron Garan, NASA'S astronaut and author of *The Orbital Perspective* feels. Ron spent over 177 days in space, looking down on the planet in his spare moments. This life-changing experience made him rethink his view of our interconnectedness as a human race. Ron shares his desire from a profound sense of hope that he believes, "If we can embrace each other, this will help propel our global society on a slightly more positive trajectory. By taking a 'big picture view,' a 'long term view' and by looking at our planet as one system. This can change our perspective and awareness making things become clear that we tend to ignore on the surface." [1]

When zooming out and looking from an orbital perspective, Ron says, "We began to realize these are symptoms of the underlying root cause which is our reluctance to acknowledge our interconnectedness." We are all a part of the same human family and what happens on one side of the world effects what happens on the other side, maybe not to the same extent, but there is a direct relationship. Ron's perspective from outer space melted away the "us" and "them" - that we are one global family, we are one species, and we have the task to take care of the land, the animals, and our children's future. There is no time to wait.

Ripple Effect

Within each of us, we carry the capacity to change the world in small ways, for better or worse. Everything we do and think affects the people in our lives, and their reactions in turn affect others.

Our thoughts and actions are like stones dropped into still waters, causing the ripples to spread and expand as they move outward. We can use the ripple effect to make a positive difference and spread waves of kindness. A healthier diet, raising our awareness, smiling at a stranger, or a thoughtful gesture can send ripples that spread among our loved ones and into our community, and finally, throughout the world. We have the power to touch the lives of everyone we come into contact with. The momentum of our influence will grow as our ripples move onward and outward. One of those ripples could become a tidal wave of love and kindness making for more peace in our world.

In Search Of Happiness

If we take a genuine look at our planet from all perspectives, ranging from the outer space to the deep oceans and seas, and look at us as humans living on the planet, we can really begin to understand how resilient and strong yet incredibly sensitive and volatile both our earth, and human body is, given the current way of living.

If we look at where happiness comes from we would start with our living conditions, community, and our health.

With a population of 7.5 billion and growing, industry and agriculture have to keep up with the demands of our busy, convenient way of living. This demand has created massive destruction on the earth and our human bodies. Let's take a truthful look at what's happening with our world and our bodies and how we can reduce our impact and also begin to thrive again in a healthy, conscious, and loving way. [2]

REVIVE OUR HEALTH = REVIVE OUR WORLD

The "Invisibles" Inside Us

To survive, we need air to breathe, water to drink, food to eat, and shelter from the elements. 50-85% of the oxygen we breathe is produced by marine plants. 97% of the earth's water supply is contained in the ocean and 30% of carbon dioxide emissions produced by humans are absorbed by the ocean. We are now producing nearly 300 million tons of plastic every year, half of which is for single use. More than 8 million tons of plastic are dumped into the ocean. Scientists agree that there's oxygen from ocean plants in every breath we take. [3]

Most of the earth's oxygen comes from tiny ocean plants called phytoplankton that live near the water's surface and drift with the currents. Measurements from the most contaminated regions of the world's oceans show that the mass of plastics exceeds that of plankton six fold. Today, plastics (phthalates) accumulate in garbage dumps and landfills and are sullying the world's oceans in ever greater quantity. They move up the ocean food chain and we ingest them. [4]

Despite the scourge of discarded plastics and the health risks these substances pose, Rolf Halden, associate professor in the School of Sustainable Engineering at Arizona State University and assistant director of the department of environmental biotechnology at the Biodesign Institute is "optimistic that society can begin to make wiser choices and develop more sustainable products, formed from biodegradable, non-toxic chemical building blocks."

New forms of polymer made from renewable materials that are digestible by microorganisms are being explored. Plastics and their additives can come in through our skin's absorption of cosmetics, toiletries, polyvinyl chloride (PVC) water pipes, detergents, pesticides, and foods. We also can inhale them from airborne adhesives, building materials, school / business supplies, furnishings, and toys. They are inside virtually all of us and are present in our blood and urine in measurable amounts. These chemicals are highly toxic and have a wide range of chronic effects, including endocrine disruption which can alter metabolic function in the body and act on estrogen pathways, which in humans, has been associated with such varied effects as decreased sperm count, endometriosis, insulin resistance, birth defects, immune system suppression, developmental problems in children, and cancer. There is no end to the tricks that endocrine disruptors can play on our bodies. They increase the production of certain hormones and decrease production of others, imitate hormones, interfere with hormone signaling, tell cells to die prematurely, compete with essential nutrients, bind to essential hormones, and accumulate in organs that produce hormones. [5]

The endocrine system refers to the collection of glands of an organism that secrete hormones directly into the circulatory system to be carried towards distant target organs. The major endocrine glands include the pineal gland, pituitary gland, pancreas, ovaries, testes, thyroid gland, parathyroid gland, hypothalamus, gastrointestinal tract, and adrenal glands. [6]

Food: Food is defined as any nutritious substance that people or animals eat or drink, or that plants absorb, in order to maintain life and growth. In order to thrive we need clean foods unadulterated, pure, and packed full of naturally occurring vitamins and minerals, from the closest source linked to nature. Today, food is not what it is supposed to be. Majority of it is grown in unnatural conditions with herbicides and pesticides. Additional hormones are introduced, and the processing leaves little to no nutrients.

Oxford Martin School researchers have found that the food system is responsible for more than a quarter of all greenhouse gas emissions, while unhealthy diets and high body weight are among the greatest contributors to premature mortality. [7] A global switch to diets that rely less on meat and focus more on fruit and vegetables could save up to 8 million lives by 2050, reduce greenhouse gas emissions by two thirds, and lead to healthcare-related savings and avoided climate damages of 1.5 trillion United States Dollars. [8] Sadly, a staggering 80% of foods are also now contaminated with a chemical called glyphosate (Roundup weed killer) that are not only damaging the earth of living organisms but are also damaging the living organisms within us. Glyphosate (N-phosphonomethylglycine), the active ingredient in the herbicide Roundup®, is the main herbicide in use today in the United States and increasingly throughout the world, in agriculture and in lawn maintenance. Eighty percent of genetically modified crops, particularly corn, soy, canola, cotton, sugar beets, and most recently alfalfa, are specifically targeted towards the introduction of genes resistant to glyphosate, and are now "Roundup Ready."

Just how corn is mass produced, soy, canola meal, and alfalfa are some of the largest grown crops to feed animals. They are some of the most widely used protein sources in animal feed for livestock, poultry, and fish. Approximately 43% of a canola seed is oil. What remains is canola meal that is used as an ingredient in animal feed. Canada is the largest single country producer of canola. According to the ISAAA, 97.5% of the canola grown in Canada last year was genetically modified. The pervasiveness of GMOs in animal feed, also makes it challenging for organic producers to secure an uncontaminated organic feed. This is a challenge that will continue to grow if GMO crops are allowed to continue their land cover growth as a result of limited supply, increasing the risk of irreversible cross-contamination.

Without strictly enforced labeling laws, consumers are being deceived into thinking they are not contributing to the consumption and production of GMOs. However, the statistics show that GMOs are hidden in our everyday foods and consumed by the animals that produce the meat, eggs, and dairy products that Americans consume in vast quantities. [9]

Glyphosate Inside Us: Mother's milk is the very first lifeline a baby is given to survive in this world where a baby is supposed to receive all the necessary protein, amino acids, and all the bioavailable vitamins and minerals for healthy growth and development. [10]

Unfortunately, with the way food is controlled and contaminated now, the news is so saddening. Research now indicates that breast milk contains extremely dangerous levels of glyphosate. The levels of glyphosate found in breast milk testing showed 76 micrograms per liter (ug/l) to 166 ug/l, which is 760 to 1600 times higher than the European Drinking Water Directive allows for individual pesticides. They are however less than the 700 ug/l maximum contaminant level (MCL) for glyphosate in the U.S., which was decided upon by the U.S. Environmental Protection Agency (EPA) based on the now seemingly false premise that glyphosate was not bioaccumulative. Glyphosate disrupts the gut microbiota leading to the overgrowth of pathogens and inflammatory bowel disease. It also negatively impacts the brain, disrupts the reproductive system, and may be a critical factor in autism, anorexia, autoimmune dysfunction, and many other disruptions in the body. [11, 12]

In fact, researchers from the University of California's San Diego School of Medicine found that human exposure to glyphosate has increased approximately 500% since 1994, when Monsanto introduced its genetically modified Roundup Ready crops in the United States. New scientific evidence shows that probable harm to human health could begin at ultra-low levels of glyphosate e.g. 0.1 parts per billions (ppb). Popular foods such as Cheerios tested for glyphosate measured between

289.47 ppb and 1,125.3 ppb. With the rise of chemicals in our food all around us and inside us, it's no wonder we are seeing a world full of depression, fatigue, anger, disease, and premature death. [13] Educating ourselves deeply can be the answer to our survival and the earth we live in today.

Our World Within: If you're wondering how the bacteria in our digestive tract could possibly be connected to our mind, it's time to meet your "second brain," the gut. With the exposure to environmental toxins, we are seeing a destruction of our healthy gut bacteria. And a gut that isn't fortified by billions of probiotics can get out of balance and overrun with yeast and bad bacteria, which produce chemicals and by-products. If you don't have enough of the good guys standing guard, the barrier can become "leaky" and allow toxins into your bloodstream that negatively affect our brain. This leads to brain fog and memory problems which in turn affect every aspect of your professional and personal life.

> If you're wondering how the bacteria in our digestive tract could possibly be connected to our mind, it's time to meet your "second brain," the gut.

Our gut and brain are inextricably linked; a disruption in either one has the capacity to seriously affect the other. Your gut bacteria produces more than 90% of all the serotonin (the "happy" chemical that plays a role in everything from mood, appetite, and sleep) in your body! The human body is colonized by a large number of microbes coexisting peacefully with their host. The most colonized site is thegastrointestinal tract (GIT). More than 70% of all the microbes in the human body are in the colon. The microbiota is essential for the development of a functional immune system. [14]

The probiotics in our gut communicate with our brain via the vagus nerve which runs from our head all the way down to our abdomen. The good news is that a lot of this communication flows up - beneficial bacteria sends mind-boosting chemicals and messages to the brain that improve our memory and cognitive function.

Healing Our Gut

There's nothing more uncomfortable than being bloated. I know this too well as this was me my whole life, but thankfully, I have turned the corner and don't get that uncomfortable bloating anymore. When we detox environmental toxins and parasites from our body and take a break from processed foods and animal products, we release pressure from the planet and our body. An easy start can be to introduce prebiotics and probiotics into our daily lives.

Prebiotics are natural indigestible fibers we get from plant-based food that probiotics use to flourish and grow. Probiotics are good bacteria or living organisms just like those found naturally in our gut. These living organisms help change or repopulate intestinal bacteria to balance gut flora. This functional component can boost immunity and overall health. Sadly, these are destroyed with antibiotics and other environmental chemicals that we get exposed to through our food and life. Now, one of the biggest destructions we are seeing is from the glyphosate levels in our food.

Prebiotics and probiotics work synergistically, thus making them a dynamic duo! Your digestive system must be able to break down food as well as aid in absorption and the assimilation of your food. This is how probiotics and prebiotics work together to balance digestion and any issues linked to poor digestion.

A healthy inner ecosystem full of healthy microflora plays a critical role in assimilating and retaining minerals. Minerals feed our adrenals so that we can build energy. In order to get the benefits of minerals in our body, we have to digest them from the mineral-rich foods we eat. Some yummy probiotics foods and drinks are sauerkraut, kombucha, and kimchi from a good organic source just to name a few.

Prebiotics, or foods containing inulin, are spirulina, which is a marine algae. Also, medicinal mushrooms like shiitake, maitake, and reishi are excellent. Organic garlic, organic chicory root, organic apple cider vinegar and honey (look for glyphosate free honey), organic leeks, bananas, Jerusalem artichoke, dandelion greens, organic rice bran solubles are all great ways to support your digestion and improve gut health.

Parasites: Parasites can live in the intestines for years without causing symptoms. When they do start affecting you, symptoms include the following: disrupted sleep, abdominal pain, diarrhea, nausea or vomiting, gas or bloating, dysentery (loose stools containing blood and mucus), rash or itching around the rectum or vulva, stomach aches, feeling tired, weight loss, and passing a worm in your stool. Doing a gentle parasite cleanse three times a year for the whole family can be really relieving and beneficial.[15] I do not recommend a parasite cleanse for pregnant women or nursing mums as you don't want to detox this into your baby.

DETOX - PROTECT - THRIVE

We clean and protect our cars and our homes so they stay bug free and last a long time through all the seasons and the years. We spend countless hours and money researching the best education for our children.

When we can clean, balance and protect our bodies, and deeply research our food source - how it is grown, what happens to it in the growth process, who controls its growth and production, and what it will do to us and our children when we ingest it - we will be in a much more conscientious and healthy state of being as global citizens. The conscious choices we make now will affect our world for years to come. They will teach our children cellular intelligence and how to feel great and energized through nature's gifts. We can save money now because our bodies are balanced and satisfied on less, and making a conscious effort to choose health and well-being over artificial and processed gunk will help us save money in the future for our health.

Making sustainable and bioavailable choices will also create and teach our children sustainability for the planet that they will be living on with their children long after we are gone. It's our responsibility to leave that wisdom for them. The gift of incredible health global consciousness, and balance are some of the greatest gifts we can offer them.

True Balance

The potential hydrogen or pH balance of our blood is a good indicator of our overall health. Human blood stays in a very narrow pH range right around 7.35 to 7.45. Below or above this range may indicate symptoms and disease. If blood pH moves too much below 6.8 or above 7.8, cells stop functioning, and the person dies. The body has to have a balanced pH like most living things on earth, or it does not function correctly. The alkaline level is very important because research has already proven that disease cannot survive in an alkaline state and instead thrives in an acidic environment. The truth is everyone has different nutrient requirements, but we all share one thing in common - we need to have alkaline blood to stay healthy.

Making sustainable and bioavailable choices will also create and teach our children sustainability for the planet...

An acidic environment will decrease the body's ability to absorb minerals and other nutrients, decrease the energy production in the cells, decrease the body's ability to repair damaged cells, decrease the body's ability to detoxify heavy metals, make tumor cells thrive, and make the body more susceptible to fatigue and illness. Most processed or junk foods are acidic. These include soft drinks, beer, coffee, candy, artificial sweeteners, cakes, and pastries made from white flour, foods high in sugar and / or sodium, sweetened yogurt, and fried foods. Plus, they cost the planet a lot of energy. [16]

Alkaline For A Super Life

Most of you reading this probably know it's healthy to drink warm lemon water, alkaline water, apple cider vinegar, and fresh-pressed green juice. Sure, they all improve your body's detox abilities, boost your immune system, and give you a mega dose of much needed nourishment. However, all these benefits occur because each of these drinks help raise your body's pH, turning your system from acidic to alkaline. Below are a few surprising foods that are alkaline and also wonderful for the whole family to enjoy. Please make sure you know your source is organic, non GMO, and free of chemicals.

Spirulina, raw almonds, broccoli, pink salt, chard, cucumber, endive, fennel, wheatgrass, kale, parsley, kelp, spinach, sprouts, sprouted beans, arugula, avocado, basil, bee pollen, beetroot, cabbage, celery, chia, chives, cilantro, escarole, figs, garlic, ginger, green beans, lemon, lettuce, Lima beans, lime, mustard greens, navy beans, okra, onion, peppers, quinoa, radish, red onion, scallion, spring greens, artichoke, asparagus, avocado oil, Brussel sprouts, buckwheat, carrot, cashew nuts, cauliflower, chestnuts, coconut (flesh, milk, water, and oil), fava beans, flax oil, grapefruit, herbs, spices, lentils, peas, pomegranate, pumpkin, rhubarb, summer squash, winter squash, sweet potato, and watercress. [17] This is a bounty of options to stay alkaline.

Spirulina - The Magic Algae: As an ecologically-sound, nutrient-rich dietary supplement, spirulina is being investigated to address food security and malnutrition, and as dietary support in long-term space flight or Mars missions. Spirulina can be used for lower land and water needs to produce protein and energy, instead of constantly relying on livestock as a dominant source of protein. [18]

Spirulina contains so much chlorophyll which carries oxygen into the body, it is extremely powerful for detoxification, the removal of harmful minerals, metals, and toxic substances from the cells and organs of the body, including mercury, which is commonly used as an amalgam for fillings in tooth cavities. Mercury fillings in teeth are cumulative toxic poisons and should be removed for health.

Spirulina is one of the most balanced and complete single sources of dietary minerals, and, therefore, including adequate amounts of spirulina in our daily diet will provide considerable benefits towards our optimal health, vitality, and well-being. It contains the 8 essential amino acids we need for survival and also the non-essential amino acids.

It also contains a large variety of naturally occurring vitamins and mineral such as biotin, calcium, vitamin B12, folic acid, inositol, iron, magnesium, niacin, pantothenic acid, phosphorous, potassium, vitamin B6, riboflavin, B2, selenium, thiamin (B1), vitamin E, and zinc.

Benefits Of Spirulina:
- Boosts "good microbes" in the digestive system, which in turn boosts our immune system
- Detoxifies the liver, organs, tissues and bowels from accumulated toxic substances
- Balances body pH to a naturally alkaline state
- Beneficial against anemia
- Cleans teeth and gums, sore throat, and mouth ulcers
- Reduces inflammatory pain
- Helps ease the symptoms of asthma
- Improves milk production in nursing women
- Helpful for post-nasal drip
- Greatly reduces or eliminates halitosis (bad breath)
- Increases red blood cell counts
- Helps regulate blood sugar levels
- Transports iron to the vital organs
- Helps to improve hepatitis
- Helps improve conditions of varicose veins
- May reduce the ability of cancerous substances to bind with DNA

Yet another very valuable component of spirulina, found in high concentration is the antioxidant superoxide dismutase (SOD). SOD belongs to a group of enzymes that repairs cellular damage caused by the most abundant free radical superoxide, which contributes towards aging. SOD behaves as a catalyst in this process which converts SOD into oxygen and hydrogen peroxide. SOD also functions as a powerful anti-inflammatory, neutralizing agent against free radical environmental toxins like phthalates, herbicides, pesticides, carbon dioxide that give rise to the signs of aging. As an anti-aging antioxidant, superoxide dismutase is 3500 times more powerful than vitamin C.

In eradicating extreme poverty and hunger - the U.N. Millennium Development Goal #1 - sustainable and long term solutions are essential. These are imperative not only in emergency situations but also as an investment in a productive society to make a change in people's everyday lives. How can society end poverty and achieve prosperity if its children are underdeveloped, mentally unwell, or too weak to attend school? One such sustainable solution is spirulina, which can serve as a vital source of nutrition, and it is extremely affordable.

UNDERSTANDING OUR HORMONES

Don't Worry, Be Happy

With the pressures of life, low nutrient value in our foods, high exposure to chemicals, less exercise, more screen time, and poor sleep, it is no wonder our hormones and our moods are all over the place.

Serotonin: Often known as the "happy hormone" because of its unique quality to regulate moods, it also plays a critical and perhaps lesser known role in everything from the formation of blood clots to enhancing our bone density in addition to having an effect on appetite, learning, memory, mood, social behavior, sexual desire and function, and temperature regulation.

Serotonin is a chemical, 90% of which is located on our gut, our second brain. It is especially active in constricting smooth muscles, transmitting impulses between nerve cells, regulating cyclic body processes, and contributing to well-being and happiness.[19] As mentioned above, becoming best friends with and loving our gut by cleaning it out and feeding it plenty of prebiotics and probiotics are sure fire ways to become a more fun person to be around. There are also some other ways we can increase our happy hormone.

Fun Ways To Increase Serotonin: Laughing is one of the easiest ways to increase the levels of serotonin and enhance the feeling of wellness. It is a natural relaxant and quickly reduces the levels of stress-related hormones. Laughter works as a mild antidepressant as it releases "feel good" endorphins and serotonin, which give the body pain relieving effects and provide the mind with a feeling of well-being boosting optimism, self-confidence, and feelings of self-worth. Massage is wonderful as we all know, and being a massage therapist myself, I love to receive a massage and definitely know why. A study researched the effects of massage on babies of depressed mothers. They massaged infants aged one to three months old, twice a week for a duration of fifteen minutes for six consecutive weeks. The infants' serotonin jumped 34%.[20]

Another good way to increase serotonin production is through physical exercise. Being physically active triggers the release of serotonin in the brain. Furthermore, it improves your muscle flexibility, and the increase in strength and endurance will help your body to cope better with anxiety attacks. It decreases the danger of heart problems in combination with high blood pressure as well as the likelihood of side effects such as muscle aches, making it easier for you to fall asleep at the end of the day and sleep deeply. Production of serotonin is closely linked to the availability of vitamin B6 and the amino acid tryptophan. If our diets are lacking in sufficient vitamins, we run a greater risk of serotonin deficiency. We may experience a dip in serotonin in relation to physiological causes, digestive disorders, and stress, since high levels of the stress hormone, also known as cortisol, rob us of serotonin.

When we measure our current lifestyle against all the elements necessary for the body's natural production of serotonin and add in chronic stress, one of the main causes of serotonin depletion, it's no wonder many of us suffer from depleted serotonin. Some plant-based foods that have the highest content of tryptophan are spirulina, spinach, raw watercress, raw pumpkin leaves, legumes, raw brown mushrooms such as Italian mushrooms and cremini mushrooms, raw horseradish-tree leafy tips, and raw sprouted greens, just to name a few.

Cortisol: Cortisol is known as the "stress hormone" because it is secreted during times of fear or stress, whenever your body goes into the fight or flight response. It is made in your adrenals. In the constant state of stress so commonplace today, cortisol creates chronic to severe inflammation that eventually causes premature aging and leads to an earlier death. [21] In fact, cortisol is often called "the death hormone." It suppresses another important hormone called dehydroepiadrosterone, or DHEA, the "youth" hormone.

Cortisol causes blood sugar levels to elevate, in turn leading to an acidic blood condition. Acidic blood leads to the modern lifestyle epidemics we see today such as diabetes, heart disease, and cancer. Cortisol also decreases dopamine (the hormone that help us stay alert) and serotonin (the hormone which aids in relaxation), so it becomes harder to stay in balance and keep stress in check. It also messes with our mood balance, and at the same time, it increases carbohydrate and fat cravings, which may lead us to eat more sugar, for example, in order to stimulate the low dopamine and serotonin.

Cortisol slows the body's metabolic rate by blocking the effects of many of our most important metabolic hormones, including insulin (so blood sugar levels suffer and carb cravings follow), serotonin (so we feel fatigued and depressed), growth hormone (so we lose muscle and gain fat), and the sex hormones testosterone and estrogen (so our sex drive falls and we rarely feel "in the mood" when we're stressed-out and awash in cortisol). Our sleep is affected immensely when our cortisol levels are high which reduces melatonin.

Fun Ways To Reduce Cortisol Levels
- Meditate daily
- Laughter: Smile and laugh, even when things do not go as planned. It'll help you stay the course.
- Play with animals
- Give generously
- Find your creative outlet or expression. This helps your mind relax and gives it a reprieve from day to day stressors.
- Engage in positive self-talk
- Practice gratitude
- Breathe calmly. There are tons of breathing exercises available on Youtube or www.gaia.com.
- Practice yoga, tai chi, dance, or swimming. Physical activity helps us stay healthy and also promotes restful sleep and de-stresses the mind and body.
- Book a massage treatment. It is a wonderful way to increase oxytocin (the love hormone) and calm the nervous system. Hug your loved ones more; human touch is very important to feel safe, heal, and grow.
- Go to bed earlier. It helps your body rest and reset every single day.
- Seek sunshine. Even during the winter months, it's important to prioritize getting outside in the sunlight whenever possible.
- Make an impactful change honestly and truthfully for the better.
- Dream big and believe in yourself.
- Move out of stressful jobs and relationships, and focus on all that is good and positive in your life, including your achievements.
- Surround yourself with uplifting, positive people, and stay connected with friends and your community.
- Stress is a normal and inevitable part of life, and we can manage it many times through exercise and nutrition, not instant fast food, but nutrient dense foods! One of my favorite superfoods is dark chocolate!
- Researchers found that eating 1.4 ounces of dark chocolate each day for two weeks lowered stress hormones like cortisol and catecholamines and can also lower blood pressure and improve mood. This only applies to dark chocolate. Look for those with at least 70% cocoa. The higher the percentage, the bitter—and better—it is. So keep on snacking! Science has you covered.

Adaptogens For Stress Relief: Adaptogenic herbs are unique from other substances in their ability to balance endocrine hormones and the immune system. They are the only natural substances able to help the body maintain optimal homeostasis. They increase the general capacity of the human body to adapt to stress and they increase resistance to disease. Adaptogens are safe, yet effective choices for building energy and fortunately they are abundantly grown in the earth's garden.

Some amazing adaptogens are ashwagandha, ginseng, medicinal mushrooms like cordyceps, reishi, chaga, rhodiola, eleutherococcus. rhodiola rosea, maca and holy basil just to name a few. [22]

Aloe Vera is another incredible adaptogen and magic superfood. It contains fatty acids, enzymes, amino acids, vitamins, minerals, and other substances. Its properties are beneficial for stress relief and proper digestion. It ensures better nutrient absorption and also eliminates harmful elements through smooth excretion. [23]

Benefits of Aloe Vera:
- Halts the growth of cancer tumors
- Lowers high cholesterol
- Boosts the oxygenation of your blood
- Eases inflammation and arthritis pain
- Protects the body from oxidative stress
- Prevents kidney stones and protects the body from oxalates
- Alkalizes the body
- Reduces ulcers, IBS, Crohn's disease and other digestive disorders
- Reduces high blood pressure
- Accelerates healing from physical burns and radiation burns
- heals the intestines and lubricates the digestive tract
- Stabilizes blood sugar
- Prevents and treats candida infections
- Functions as nature's own "sports drink" for electrolyte balance, making common sports drinks obsolete.
- Boosts cardiovascular performance and physical endurance.
- Speeds recovery from injury or physical exertion.
- Hydrates the skin, accelerates skin repair.

Wheatgrass - Nature's Mood Enhancer

According to a 2014 literature review in the *Asian Journal of Pharmaceutical Technology and Innovation*, not only does wheatgrass boost the adrenal system thanks to its vitamin K and magnesium content, thus helping your body cope with stress, it is also rich in iron. And according to the Mayo Clinic, iron deficiency can cause fatigue, which worsens mood and makes you feel blasé and unenthused. The study showed that keeping iron levels balanced is crucial for those suffering from depression, and the iron in wheatgrass is one way to contribute to this. [24]

Wheatgrass is 70% chlorophyll, which increases the level of oxygen in the blood, which allows harmful toxins to flow out of our body. Its high phenolic content allows it to bind to chelated metal ions in the colon and liver. [25, 26] Wheatgrass prevents tooth decay, stimulates the immune system, supports the lungs by healing scars from gases, cleanses the liver, improves digestion as it contains loads of fiber and b-complex vitamins, reduces fatigue, eliminates body odor, stabilizes lipid levels, fights radiation, slows aging, stabilizes blood sugar levels, and helps increase fertility. Wheatgrass is a source of potassium and protein (less than one gram per 28 grams). It also has a high amount of biologically active enzymes and amino acids as well as dietary fiber, vitamin A, vitamin C, vitamin E (alpha tocopherol), vitamin K, thiamin, riboflavin, niacin, vitamin B6, pantothenic acid, iron, zinc, copper, manganese, and selenium.

Melatonin - Sweet Dreams Do Come True

Our body has its own internal clock that controls our natural sleep cycle. In part, our body clock controls how much melatonin our body makes. Normally, melatonin levels begin to rise in the mid to late evening, remain high for most of the night, and then drop in the early morning hours. Melatonin is produced by various tissues in the body although the major source is the pineal gland in the brain. The production and release of melatonin from the pineal gland occurs with a clear daily (circadian) rhythm, with peak levels occurring at night. Melatonin is carried by the circulation from the brain to all areas of the body. Tissues expressing proteins called receptors specific for melatonin are able to detect the peak in circulating melatonin at night and this signals to the body that it is nighttime. The level of circulating melatonin can be detected in samples of urine. [27] There are a number of factors that influence our melatonin production such as stress, lack of exposure to natural light during the day, increased exposure to light at night (often from television, phones, computers, and clocks), working a night shift, travel and time zone changes (also known as jet lag), lack of sleep due to various factors (for e.g. parents up through the night with an infant/child), leaky gut, nutrient deficiencies, inflammation, and parasites.

Increasing self-care can be challenging after tending to our children and our jobs; however, it can be a powerful way to increase melatonin. Scheduling in a gentle yoga class, practicing weekly meditation, or treating yourself to a massage when you can is very important for reducing cortisol and increasing serotonin and oxytocin to reverse the catabolic effects on our bodies.

Here are a few other effective ways to increase melatonin production:
- Exercising for a minimum of twenty to thirty minutes a day
- Avoid having too big of a meal or sugar hours before bed
- Relaxing before bed: try a warm bath, reading, or another relaxing routine.
- Creating an ambience conducive for good and restful sleep: avoid bright lights and loud sounds, keep the room at a comfortable temperature, and don't watch TV or have a computer in your bedroom.

Tart Cherry: The juicy secret? Tart cherry juice, the antioxidant-rich liquid that's increasingly being hailed as an answer to pain, swelling, sleeplessness, and anti-aging. [28] Tart cherry concentrate from the Montmorency cherry is nature's only naturally occurring form of melatonin and is incredible to relieve oxidative stress. It is best taken just before your brush your teeth, turn off all lights, phones, and computers, and roll into bed. You will get a deep R.E.M. sleep which is crucial for putting the body into a healing state.

Montmorency cherries contain up to 13.5 nanograms (ng) of melatonin per gram of cherries, more than is normally found in the blood. Melatonin is by far the most potent of the antioxidants, much more so than vitamins C, E, and A. The reason: Melatonin is soluble both in fat and water and can therefore enter some cells that vitamins cannot. Even with the small study covering a short time period, researchers found marked differences between the experimental and control groups. Irrespective of the dose, blood and urine samples revealed more uric acid was leaving the body, and C-reactive protein levels were lower. This signaled a reduced risk for gout, a form of arthritis that can cause severe attacks of intense pain and swelling. Cherries have been revered for their anti-inflammatory properties for years. Drinking even small quantities of Montmorency tart cherry juice has been linked to decreased levels of uric acid in the blood along with a key biomarker for inflammation, known as C-reactive protein, according to a pair of new studies.

By choosing to take conscious action to decrease the stressors in our lives, clean out toxins, and nourish ourselves at the cellular level, we will sleep better at night, increase happiness, reduce anxiety, and truly become the change we wish to see in the world. We can live vibrantly, lovingly, and begin to make our dreams come true. We begin to think clearer, raise our awareness, and our vibration, hence creating an abundance of enough energy to support our family, friends, our community, and the future of the planet. When we can consciously change our thoughts and actions, we leave that legacy of wisdom for our children to continue on in our footsteps.

THANK YOU

In complete gratitude, I thank you Ky-Lee Hanson, for creating this opportunity to share my voice and knowledge alongside these other intelligent beautiful women.

I give thanks and dedicate this piece to my sweet family, friends, community, and the world.

I give thanks and honor to my incredible, supportive husband Aaron, for always being a huge part of my growth and a fun loving pillar of strength. It's been beautiful to witness you as a gentle and intelligent father to our son, Levi.

Thank you Mom, Dad, Pete, Caron, Gene, and Iris for always believing in me and supporting through this passionate path. I love you guys so much.

Levi, mommy and daddy wished for you over many moons. To this day, since you were born, I know that you are by far, and will forever be, my greatest teacher. It is for you and all your little friends I forge the way to make a difference on this planet so you can live in abundance and purity on this earth with your children and grandchildren.

May we all bring love and harmony into the world and come together to make a massive wave of positive change for our children of the future.

~ Rebecca Hall

A TOXIC AGENDA

YOU DO NOT HAVE TO LIVE LIFE CAPTIVE
TO SICK CARE. YOU CAN OPT OUT
AND LIVE LIFE TRULY HEALTHY, NATURALLY.

by Meghan Rose

(ret.) Infectious Disease Registered Nurse, RN
Certified Vaccine Education Specialist

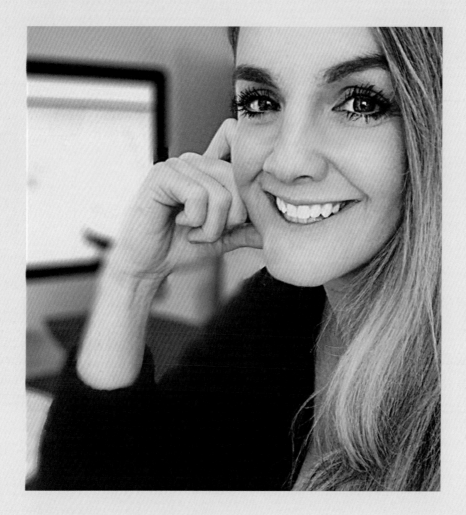

Meghan Rose

Meghan is a former infectious disease registered nurse turned internet entrepreneur, holistic health enthusiast, blogger, and activist.

She lives on the east coast with her husband Keith and her five beautiful children. She is passionate about her faith, and homeschooling, and is an activist for medical freedom and vaccine education. She specializes in coaching women through a cellular cleansing nutritional system and offers free consultations on vaccine education and reducing toxic chemicals in the home.

fb: thevaccinefreemom

When I was growing up, I always knew that I wanted a career where I would be helping people in a major way. My parents instilled in me from a very young age that I could do anything that I set my mind to, and I have always been very empathetic, so it is no surprise that I chose a career in nursing. The first three years of my nursing career, I worked in an infectious disease unit, but my life would take a drastically different turn where I would be able to help people on a totally different level. It may seem silly that I went to school for four years only to work for three years, but the way that I look at it, we have one shot at this life. And when we feel our hearts pulling us so strongly toward something, in a direction where our fire inside of us is truly burning with passion, we absolutely need to follow that instinct, to embrace it with every fiber of our being.

"The doctor of the future will give no medicine but will interest his patients in the care of the human frame, in diet and in the cause and prevention of disease."

~ THOMAS EDISON

I am blessed to be the mother of five beautiful children: four boys and one girl. My oldest son has always struggled in a school setting. He had trouble respecting personal-space boundaries, some obsessive-compulsive tendencies, hyperactivity, and anxiety. For many years, his teachers urged me to have him evaluated for attention deficit hyperactivity disorder (ADHD), and for just as long, I brushed them off. ADHD was a true rarity while I was growing up, as were all chronic illnesses (especially in children). During my school years, I knew one person with asthma and one person with ADHD. Food allergies were practically unheard of, as were autism-spectrum disorders. So in my mind, the ADHD possibility was, for lack of a better term, ridiculous… a made up term for kids who had extra energy because they didn't get outdoors enough during the school-day. I believed my son was simply "being a boy," who would outgrow this behavior as he got older. However, my beliefs did not come to fruition, and just the opposite happened for my boy. As he got older, these tendencies got worse.

After years of frustration from teachers and at home, years of hoping and praying things would get better with no luck, I was at my wit's end. It wasn't fair for me to withhold medication from him if there was truly something going on that he had no control over. I made the long-overdue appointment with his pediatrician for an evaluation. He was diagnosed with ADHD and then prescribed a medication. I was assured the medication was safe and effective with side effects being very rare. We were relieved to finally have some answers and to finally have a solution. He started his medication the next day, and it didn't take long at all to notice a very positive difference in him in school. He was able to sit still. He didn't have outbursts, and he was, in general, much happier. We were ecstatic.

Things seemed to calm down for a while, but slowly, we noticed some of his old behaviors starting to come back. I checked with his pediatrician, who assured us that this was completely normal. He told us that sometimes people's bodies adjust to medication and then require a higher dosage for therapeutic effect. Having implicit trust in his pediatrician, we agreed to increase his dosage. Again, we saw positive results, and again, those results were short-lived. At about this time, in addition to the very obvious fact that his medication was not working again, my son also started to experience some side effects: loss of appetite (getting him to eat was practically impossible), trouble sleeping (literally only sleeping for two to three hours at night), dry mouth, and heart palpitations.

We made another trip to his pediatrician, who recommended increasing his dosage one last time before trying something different, and in addition, he also recommended other medications for his decreased appetite and sleep. I was reluctant because of the side effects but had implicit trust in his doctor, so I agreed to it. We increased the dose and saw the usual improvement in attention; however, his side effects continued to get worse.

This time, I was not comfortable increasing his medication dose, but what I didn't know was that he couldn't function in class without it. I felt so torn, and it was at that point that one of my old high school friends asked me if I had ever thought of making changes in his diet to help him. I had always scoffed at "natural" cures before, but I was desperate and willing to try anything to help my son. I began researching obsessively.

It is AMAZING what information you can learn if you are simply willing to be open-minded. My entire life, I sneered at the holistic health community, thinking they were some sort of crazy, but what I learned was to put aside my preconceived notions and actually examine this information for myself. What I learned literally blew my mind. I was fascinated and outraged all at the same time. I learned that for many years, decades even, we, as a society, have been duped into thinking that we are safe and protected by some power that is looking out for our health. That is simply not true. I learned that if we truly want to be healthy, we need to be our own detectives and advocates. I took what I learned, and I applied that knowledge into my family's life. With the changes that I made, I was able to successfully help my son control his ADHD, his obsessive compulsive disorder (OCD), and his anxiety without pharmaceutical medication. In addition, I was able to change the health of our entire family. This was a pivotal time in my life... a time where, instead of choosing to go back for a master's degree in nursing, I chose to pursue something that lit my fire like nothing else ever has, other than my faith... and that is educating people on exactly everything that I have learned: Helping families reduce their chemical body burden and helping them live healthily, naturally.

We should not have to be our own detectives or our own advocates. If there is lack of safety data, or if data is remotely questionable, products should not be allowed to be distributed to the masses. And until we DO have a government or agency that is assuring the absolute safety of the food we eat and the personal care products we use, we DO have to be advocates. We HAVE to be a voice for our children, and we have an obligation to future generations to educate others and to leave this world as a place that is safe for them to live in. Making changes can be overwhelming, but knowledge is power. Together, we can make little changes, which when multiplied by many, can create massive shifts and pave the way for revolutionary change for our children and our world. Let's look more in depth into a couple of these issues.

Food Matters

Our food "system" is not what it used to be, and this topic has enough information and history to fill an entire book by itself. My goal is inspire the reader to do more research on her own. So let's start here. Food was the first place that I started researching, and our diet was the first area to experience this lifestyle change, in a life-changing manner. I learned that children with ADHD did very well without dairy, gluten, and artificial colors. Inspired by that article and by some health blogs, I took those recommendations a step further and went completely "clean" and organic with our food. Even though my son was not on medication, I noticed a dramatic improvement in his behavior. I, also, for the first time in my life, was not yo-yo-ing with my weight. I was able to maintain a very health weight without trying. My skin and energy also improved. How did this happen? It happened because what we eat matters, and eating healthily, that is, eating to fuel, nourish, and heal our body properly, is the single most important thing we can do to reduce our risk of developing disease. So why is it, with all of our technological and medical advancements today, that we have a generation that is chronically sick from a myriad of ailments? Today, an estimated 15-35% of children are suffering from chronic illness. [1] One in sixty-eight children are being diagnosed with autism [2], and cancer is the number one leading cause of death by disease among children. [3] These rates are alarming and disturbing, and while experts can't pinpoint one specific cause, there is a consensus that the majority of these issues (about 90%) are caused by environmental issues. So, it is something WE are doing.

Let's look a little more closely at our food system.

> we have an obligation to future generations to educate others and to leave this world as a place that is safe for them to live in.

GMOs

You have probably heard of the term GMO, which stands for genetically modified organism. A GMO is just literally a species of animal or plant whose genes have been altered in a laboratory setting. The first GMO patent was issued by the FDA in 1980, but GMO crops didn't become widely used until the late 1990s. [4] Numerous studies have provided evidence between GM food and a multitude of health issues. One of the first studies conducted on GMO safety was funded by the British Government and conducted at the Rowett Institute in Scotland. In this study, rats were divided into three groups and fed a balanced diet, but each group was fed a different kind of potato. One group was fed GMO potatoes, one group was fed organic potatoes, and the last group was fed non-GMO potatoes with pesticides. The only group of rats that got sick were the ones who were fed GMO potatoes. Since that study was published in the prestigious *Lancet* publication, many more studies have been published that have shown GMOs proliferate the gastrointestinal tract, cause immune system disturbance, interfere with organ development, and may be linked to tumors. Sixty-four countries around the world have GMO labeling laws in place, and thirty countries completely banned them altogether (this has increased from 26 in 2013). Despite the potential for adverse health reactions, according to the FDA, between 88-90% of all corn, soybean and cotton crops are still genetically modified today. And according to a 2015 ABC News Survey, 93% of Americans want genetically modified food to be labeled, the United States has yet to enact labeling laws. Few individual states have signed and implemented individual mandatory labeling laws, only to have them overridden by a federal law in 2016.

Regardless of whether or not labels are mandated, with some simple education, avoiding GMOs doesn't have to be difficult. Here are some quick facts and need-to-knows:

Different types of GMOs

BT Toxin: These crops create their own pesticide, BT Toxin, which literally makes the stomach of the insect eating it, explode.

Roundup Ready: Roundup Ready crops are made to withstand copious amounts of the weed-killing herbicide, Roundup. Glyphosate, which is Roundup's active ingredient (see chapter 1), has been shown to have detrimental health effects, being linked to multiple issues such as ADHD, Alzheimer's disease, autism, birth defects, cancer, celiac disease and gluten intolerance, chronic kidney disease, colitis, depression, diabetes, heart disease, hypothyroidism, inflammatory bowel disease, liver disease, ALS, multiple sclerosis, non-Hodgkin lymphoma, Parkinson's disease, infertility, miscarriage, obesity, and respiratory illnesses.

Desired Trait: These crops are genetically modified by having a desired trait injected. This is done via "promoters" that wake genes up. An example of this would increasing the color pigmentation in a red apple or green pepper to make them look more red or green respectively.

If you are unsure whether a certain product has GMOs or not, look for the non-GMO Project Verified label or the USDA Organic certification. If a product has the USDA Organic certification, it cannot, by law, contain GMOs. If a product has neither one of these labels, there is a good chance it does, in fact, contain genetically modified ingredients, especially if it contains one or more of the following ingredients, which are the most widely used:

- Soy
- Corn
- Canola
- Cotton
- Milk
- Sugar
- Aspartame
- Zucchini
- Yellow squash
- Papaya

To ensure you are getting the most nutritional value out of all of the food you are eating, connect with local farmers in your area, and ask them about their farming practices. Buy locally grown produce that is currently in season. Eating seasonally is also a good way to eat clean, nutritious food and still stay within your grocery budget. If you have to shop at a major grocery chain, stick to the outside perimeter of the store, and check the Environmental Working Group (EWG) ratings on their website for their yearly recommendations on produce that has the least and most amount of pesticide residue.

Personal Care Products

We had the nutrition part of our health down to a T and were noticing remarkable health improvements because of our lifestyle change. I recall scrolling the news headlines of the day from my phone while I was sitting in my living room nursing my then six-month-old baby while the other kids were napping.

I wasn't so much into all of the political headlines at the time, but one health headline did stop me dead in my tracks. It was titled something to the effect of

- Chemicals In Personal Care Products That Are Banned In Europe But Not in the US. Toxic shampoo? Cancer-causing anti-perspirant? I had never given a second thought to this issue, and when I was done reading, I practically needed to put my eyeballs back into my head. I ran up to my bathroom and compared ingredients in my products to that list of toxic ingredients, and every single one of my products contained at least one of those chemicals in it. I felt duped and outraged at the same time. Call me naive… but aren't we all human? If an ingredient is deemed toxic to the population in Europe, then why would it not also be deemed toxic to the population in the US? I was so confused about why this was happening, and this subject alone needs its own book. Again, my goal is to give you the information you need to reduce your chemical burden *today*. Everyone knows about the importance of nutrition, but this issue doesn't get nearly the attention it deserves. Here is the scoop:

The European Union has higher safety standards than we do here in the United States not only with food but also with personal care products. For so long, I always believed there was some "power-that-be" that was ensuring the safety of products that we put on our bodies. Our skin is our body's largest organ, and while it does create a protective barrier for some things, products we put on our skin can be absorbed directly into our bloodstream (think patch medicinal delivery systems such as the nicotine or birth control patch). Chemical usage here in the US has increased 2000% over the last fifty years with over 7,700 chemicals currently in commerce. [5] Out of that number, only 300 chemicals have ever been tested for safety. [6] Some more alarming facts - women, on average, are exposed to 168 chemicals before they even walk out the door in the morning, and a study done by the Environmental Working Group (EWG) found that babies are actually being born "pre-polluted" with over 300 chemicals found in the umbilical cord blood. [7]

So, what is a woman to do? Surely we don't all need to resort to using only apple-cider vinegar and baking soda for all of our personal care and cleaning needs? No ladies! You simply need to know what ingredients to AVOID. Nevermind all of the healthwashing that takes place today with many companies claiming that their products and ingredients are "natural" and "green." Anything that is on the front of a product is simply a clever marketing tactic! ALWAYS look at the list of ingredients!

The below list from the EWG is not comprehensive, but is a great starting point on what ingredients to avoid, and WHY.

- BHA
- Sodium borate
- Coal tar hair dyes and other coal tar ingredients (including aminophenol, di-aminobenzene, phenylenediamine)
- Formaldehyde,
- Formaldehyde releasers (bronopol, DMDM hydantoin, diazolidinyl urea, im-idzaolidinyl urea, and quaternium-15)
- Fragrance
- Methylisothiazolinone, methylchloroisothiazolinone, and benzisothiazolinone
- Oxybenzone
- Parabens (specifically propyl-, isopropyl-, butyl-, and isobutylparabens)
- PEGs/Ceteareth/Polyethylene compounds
- Phthalates
- Resorcinol
- Toluene
- Triclosan and triclocarban
- Vitamin A compounds (palmitate, retinyl acetate, retinol)

For more information on personal care safety and ingredients to avoid, check out the Environmental Working Group's cosmetic and personal care safety website at www.skindeep.org.

Environmental Impact

One topic I would be remiss not to cover is the environmental threat these toxins pose to our precious planet. These toxic chemicals have to go somewhere. When we spray our crops, many insects such as bees and butterflies come in contact with harmful toxins as well. Is it a coincidence that both types of insects are now dying off? Glyphosate, which is highly toxic and has been classified a probable carcinogen by the World Health Organization, is water soluble. It runs off into rivers and streams when it rains. Think of the same scenario when you wash your hair with a toxic shampoo to wash your hair. Where are those chemicals going? Well, they go down the drain and into water treatment facilities, where the waste will eventually end up somewhere, out of our sight and out of our mind.

However, just because we can't see these things doesn't mean we should ignore it. We have one planet to live on and one planet to leave to our future generations. Therefore, we have a moral obligation to care for it and make it more sustainable with environmentally friendly choices.

Since I began this journey into holistic health four years ago, the organic market has increased dramatically, and it is so awesome to see. Back then, I couldn't find a single non-toxic personal care product in my grocery store. Now, there are entire sections dedicated to non-toxic personal care. Organic and non-gmo food choices were few and far between. Now, you see them literally everywhere you go. This change would never have happened if there hadn't been an uprising by consumers demanding healthier and safer options. We can picket, we can protest, we can write to our congressmen, but the most effective way to be heard the loudest is to choose wisely where you spend your money. WE hold ALL of the power; we just don't give ourselves enough credit in this area sometimes! When we stop buying toxic products and food, they will have to stop making them and start making safer alternatives. Making these changes isn't hard! This natural lifestyle not only completely transformed my son's health but our entire family's life. I want this for everybody. You can do this. Your health and well-being deserve this. Our planet deserves this.

THANK YOU

First and foremost - I give glory to God for this opportunity to share my passion with so many people, and my Savior, Jesus Christ, for sustaining me through the process of balancing work, children, life, and still being able to contribute to this book. Thank you to my mom and dad for always instilling in me the belief that I can do anything I set my mind to. Thank you to my husband, Keith, for always supporting me in my endeavors and my passions - you are a good man and an example to all men everywhere. God has blessed me with you! And to my precious children - I love you more than words can ever express. You are the reason I do what I do. I will never stop fighting for you. Love, Mom.

~ Meghan Rose

LISTEN TO YOUR BODY - WHATEVER THAT MEANS...

OUR BODY CONSTANTLY SENDS US MESSAGES, WE SIMPLY HAVE TO LEARN ITS LANGUAGE.

by Ky-Lee Hanson

Nutritional Therapist, NT

KY-LEE HANSON

Bosswoman | Visionary | Creator of opportunity & motivation

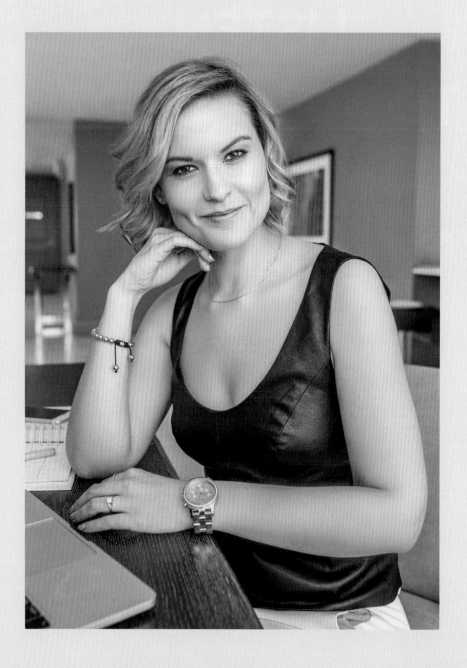

Ky-Lee Hanson is an "idea" person: always seeking deeper understanding, and providing new visions to the world. She is inquisitive, self-efficient, and self-aware. Ky-Lee creates and executes dozen of projects at a time and lends a helpful word and guidance directly to hundreds of people every week. Ky-Lee is very curious about herself, life, and people in general; she finds it all fascinating. Her studies in sociology, human behavior, stress management, nutrition, and health sciences have led her to have a deep understanding of people. She is optimistic but understands things for what they really are. Being someone who can spot potential, one of the hardest things she ever had to learn was: You can't help someone who doesn't want to help themselves.

Growing up, she had a difficult time understanding why people couldn't seem to live the lives they dreamed of. Often thinking she must be the main character in a world similar to *The Truman Show*, because nothing seemed to make sense, she always saw things differently and found it challenging to relate to people. This ended up sending her into a downward spiral in her twenties, when she felt she had no choice but to settle. She felt suppressed, limited, and angry. Ky-Lee has the ability to hyperfocus and learn things quickly. She has a power-mind, and found the true strength of life and her endless capabilities through a serious health battle in her late twenties. Ky-Lee took control and, over the years, mastered how to get her power back: mind, body, and soul. She also discovered the best way to "relate" to people is not to; instead, simply listen to understand their world for the uniqueness that it is.

Ky-Lee has formal training from Humber College in sociology, holds a professional diploma as a nutritional therapist from The Health Sciences Academy UK, and completed nutrition courses at Vanderbilt University School of Nursing, and Duke University within sports medicine. She studied nutrition, health sciences, and homeopathy at CCHM including the equivalency of first year nursing studies, and has her Reiki level 1 certification. She gravitates towards biochemistry, plant-based medicine, and food science to alleviate her ailments. Her 2019 studies include the endocannabinoid system, nutrigenetics, masculine and feminine energy balancing, and personality types.

Ky-Lee is a 4x best selling author and a successful serial entrepreneur. She thrives on creating opportunities to help people along their journey, and she excels at it. Her success came by developing the taboo art of collaborative business. Ky-Lee has an open-door policy she learned from her mom, a listening ear, and an opportunity to lock arms and take you down your *Golden Brick Road*.

WWW.GOLDENBRICKROAD.PUB | WWW.GBRSOCIETY.COM
ig: kylee.hanson.bosswoman | fb: kylee.hanson

Unfortunately in our society, we view illness as something we "own," such as "I *have* diabetes," or "I *am* anemic." We treat it as if we cannot do anything about it. We justify owning illness as normal, as part of our life, and identify *as* it. I am sorry if this is not what you want to hear, but we must acknowledge behavior and conditioning in order for us and others to live better. We can find hope in accepting many people go into complete remission, reverse illness, and drastically change their lives for the better, everyday. We won't all overcome our illnesses, but it is worth trying, isn't it? Some labels I have worn are "I am fat," "I have precancer," "I have acne," or "I am a stress case," but really, I should have been saying, "I am experiencing a deficiency or imbalance." I was never taught how to fix myself, so I accepted these states as my way of life. I honor that we can not change everything, but we DO choose how we manage it. We are given medication and / or surgery for this, that, and whatever else, but rarely are we empowered with actual knowledge of the human body, the cause and effect of what is *actually* going on. There is a fine line between health and illness; people think this line is thick, but it is not. When I was growing up, *and still to this day with all we now know*, it was as if cancer was at random selection. It is not. Sometimes things are not fair, and never is illness deserved. But it isn't always random selection. Something caused it. Maybe it is hereditary, maybe something currently untraceable happened, but there is always a cause. It is not a blame game; it is not always our fault, but an imbalance, a genetic or an epigenetic change, or compound damage, lead to the effect. While it is not hard to figure this out, and we know stress, illness, and disease are riddling our society, we are conditioned to be fine with feeling only okay. We have been conditioned to think that as long as we can get out of bed, we are good enough. Society makes us continue to plug away, while our cells are gasping for oxygen, and loads of problems are manifesting inside us. There are a lot of people in this world that are constantly a bit discolored, tired, suffering from digestive issues, have aches and pain, skin issues or sinus problems - but! That isn't an "illness" according to society, that is "common." The truth is, their body is in a constant acidic state; they are chronically sick. Constant irritability of the body, also known as an imbalance, eventually compounds. Disease is caused from cumulative damage, if we do not heal as often as we hurt, it will continue to get worse.

The illness that shaped my life was C111 cervical dysplasia. The last stage of abnormal cellular progression before cervical cancer. My doctors referred to me as having a precancer. When I was ill, it seemed that every book, and every person was telling me eating was a problem not a solution, I couldn't find resources; the only answer provided was painkillers and surgery but I saw past the passiveness and scare tactics of drug and medical pushers, to find for myself, food can also be a solution. I couldn't help but ask myself, *Should I be trusting these people on*

- EVERYthing? I logically decided: Surgeons specialize in surgery, not nutrition. I need more help.

This illness inside of me started, *well who really knows*, probably sometime as a teen. I had intense menstrual bleeding, my nutrition was terrible, and there was so much stress in my life. My dad left, there were constant money struggles, I didn't fit in, we moved cities; my boyfriend at the time sucked, I partied a lot, and I worked in fast food: long hours, poor working conditions, little stimulation and lots of consuming low quality food and sugar. My life continued like this into my twenties except that I got a good - the best - boyfriend and started to pay more attention to food. From the first time I heard about GMOs, I felt they were a bad idea. I then began researching more about factory farming, and my meat reduction phase began. At the time, I didn't have a lot of money, and I still worked in hospitality. So even though I was learning, I was not applying this new found knowledge to the level I should have been. My practice of nutrition was "convenience."

At this point, I didn't know what the "label" was for my condition. My illness got to a point where I passed out in the bath due to menstrual cramping. Another time, I was managing a restaurant and collapsed on the bathroom floor, then huddled for what felt like a day, in the corner of that dirty washroom. The pain was so intense. I was bleeding to a point that seemed like hemorrhaging. The few years leading up to this I had commonly experienced insomnia, night sweats, eczema, depression, and anxiety. I was angry and irrational, experiencing digestive issues daily: irritable bowel syndrome (IBS) and vomiting. My acne was out of control. My hair was falling out. My skin was basically green or as they call "olive" which I thought was normal for my heritage, but I was actually becoming discolored. It was all progressively happening, so I learned how to live with all these symptoms, continued to go to work, and continued to eat "affordable" foods, until it was too much. I was waking up in puddles of sweat. I remember standing at the end of the bed and telling my spouse, "Matty, this isn't normal." *Yet, I am pretty sure he was telling me this for years. But I never found doctors helpful, and I was scared. I knew something was wrong, and I tried to ignore it.* I remember feeling ashamed and embarrassed, but mostly scared. I had zero internal power to fix myself. I was tired, I was sick, and I was not knowledgeable enough about my body.

Not all women want to get an intrauterine device (IUD), and we all have our right to be unique and decide for ourselves. But for me, this was the answer. I no longer experience bleeding, only spotting, and I no longer have crippling cramps or muscle tremors, nor do I pass out from menstrual pain anymore or overheat or suffer from insomnia related to my menstrual cycle. I had all of this wrong with me which led to so much stress on my body, anemia, and malnutrition - *yes, even though I live in the western world and have always had a job* - as our society indirectly promotes deficiencies. Most of us do not know what *and in what quantities of* vitamins and minerals make up our bodies, causing us to not get what we need = malnutrition. People consume mostly yellow and white foods - bread, potatoes, rice, sugar, dairy, poultry, beer, and white wine. We do not get what we need, and most people are passive about this. We live in a go-go-go society where practical knowledge is shunned. My common lifestyle eventually accumulated into what could have been my demise.

While in the process of working with a specialist who suggested the IUD, she discovered the aggressive abnormalities in my cells. It took me years of explaining my symptoms to doctors before I got in to see the specialist. It took bleeding to the point of going in and out of consciousness for them to give me a referral, which then took another year to get in. Looking back, with just a bit of research and speaking to naturopaths, it is evident that the symptoms I was chronically experiencing were messages from my body that something serious was trying to manifest inside of me. Through my applied studies and through working with natural health practitioners, it was learned that I was estrogen dominant. This is why the IUD had such positive effect on me. It would have served me if a doctor explained this to me from the start. I can't count how many doctors did nothing but prescribe eczema cream and naproxen. These don't fix anything! Although I had extended medical coverage, I was never suggested a recommendation to talk to a dietician, or a therapist for a lifestyle / career change.

So, I had surgery in my mid-twenties. It did not work. It was the most scary day of my life, so scary that I fled to Mexico for the four months prior to surgery. I couldn't simply live normally waiting for the day to come. It just so happened that the prep and surgery fell during the week of my twenty-seventh birthday. Devastating. I made it through with just one trip back to the emergency room, monthly checkups, and a summer off work and on bed rest, only to find out the surgery didn't work. I was told I had seven months before they predicted I would have full blown cervical cancer. My doctor prepared surgery dates for me to have my cervix completely removed.

Fuck that. No way. I spent the next two weeks of my life, every waking hour, in front of the computer learning about cervical cancer, dysplasia, cellular health, what makes a cell abnormal, what makes a cell healthy, and what can I do about it. I read books, asked questions, messaged all sorts of wellness people, read medical blogs, taught myself basic biochemistry, and I then found myself working in food science and skincare. The amount of estrogen that builds up in our body from consuming animal products and the ingredients we absorb from skincare is mind boggling. I could see the working parts in food, products, and myself. It was all connected. *I am made up of the same thing as plants.* All of this empowered me; it made me stronger. I felt happy and powerful for, honestly, the first time in many years. Every bit of trust was lost for my doctor, so I got another opinion - five to be exact. I had to keep asking until I found a doctor who would tell me what I wanted to hear. I was asking, can a healthy body fix this on its own? It took five doctors telling me, "Well, we just don't know for certain," and "We won't test you again as your doctor just did." At one point, I was in a room with three doctors blatantly disregarding them. I swear if they said, "We just don't know," one more time... I truly began to question what *did* they know? This was my LIFE. Finally, they sent me to a doctor who came from Europe. It clicked that I was relentless, and although I didn't have my answer, he knew I was adamant to find it. I asked him "hypothetically" what are the chances? He replied that three out of four bodies will correct abnormal cells on their own, but in my case, with the frequency, they can't risk me being in the remaining 25%. Okay, valid. *Now we are talking.* I am finally being empowered with information on my body. I asked, what are commonalities in those three of the four? While there is not a works-for-everyone or proven method, the general knowledge is those people would have good genes, low illness history with healthy lifestyle habits, be a non smoker, and likely are active. Okay, I asked him what was the longest amount of time he could give me before I had to go under the knife? I was given three months.

Three Months To Change My Life So I Could Save My Life

Milk was the first thing to go. A vegan diet made up 95% of my meals. I took graviola and indole-3-carbinol daily along with high quality pro and prebiotics, folic acid, vitamin B12, and many more. My pantry had one shelf full of vitamins, in rows based on how many to take per day. I was up to about forty supplements per day. I ate veggies, all the time. I drank smoothies every morning. We cooked at home, keeping on top of ingredient control. We ordered farm fresh organic food, the most expensive I could find. I was spending $1000 a month on my health. Matty and I would do Crossfit in our living room almost daily, and we got YMCA gym passes. I ran out all my anger towards illness on a treadmill.

I got better. The three months passed, and I was ecstatic to get the biopsy done. My empowered, educated, clear mind that was focused on a goal was my most powerful remedy. I knew I was better. I could feel it. If you have illness inside you, you know it is there. Don't wait like I did. I suffered because I was scared. There were zero, ZERO, abnormal cells inside my cervix, and a few that were no longer "severe" on the outside. All I needed done was a loop electrosurgical excision procedure (LEEP), NOT surgery, to have my cervix removed. If I hadn't done something about it, I wouldn't have my cervix today. But here I am, whole.

Although the doctors kept me on strict follow up (there were times in my life I was at the hospital monthly), I have never had an issue since. It has been five years. The forty supplements a day didn't last all that long; I have lots in my cupboard and have some on daily ritual, while others I take as I feel the need for them. I learned to listen and trust my body, to be one with it. I never did go back to eating red meat or poultry, nor drinking milk; however, fish, cheese, and eggs I did consume. My diet has remained mostly vegan; my skincare and household products are natural and vegan. I barely work out anymore. *I don't enjoy it much.* But I know I should and will start again.

I am neither ill, nor am I a health freak. I am me. I give my body what it needs, and when I do things that are not all that great, I fix it. I went from one extreme to the next to somewhere in the middle, not always balanced but in around there. My hair is healthy. I only get acne when I reduce the green superfoods in my life, and I am thirty-three years-old and barely have any facial wrinkles (I actually had more when I was twenty-seven-years-old and sick). There was no miracle for me. There was zero luck. It was all determination, belief, education, and mostly self will.

Our vitality, health, and well-being require us to dig deep and know who we are: mind, body, and spirit, our triggers, ailments, and constitution, all our strengths and weaknesses. Then, learn what counteracts them. I am "hypersensitive" compared to others because I understand every inch of my body. As I mentioned, it took time and serious illness, both mentally and physically, for me to realize and understand this. After all I went through, it is not surprising that I am the way I am. I know there are people out there like me and like the confused person riddled with illness that I used to be. A piece of advice I'd like to address is not related to the food you put into your body but in relation to the openness of your mind to learn and accept change. A lot of people expect a quick fix, or they will opt to continue to suffer. It does take learning, and learning is always uncomfortable in the beginning. It's hard! But you are capable. Just as illness is cumulative, so is well-being. The more we continue to add good into our life, the less room there is for the bad things. If you let it get out of control like I did, you need to do some serious damage control. Go intense about health for three months. Matty and I have a three month rule of thumb. Anything we want to learn or get good at, we do for three months straight. It is the reason I know a wealth of knowledge; I dive into four new things every year.

When I speak about investment into health and how I was spending $1000 a month, I am not pushing any sort of product on you; I actually like to encourage education. To this day, I don't know if everything I did was necessary, but at the time, it was worth it. Learning and trying new things shocked my mind and body in positive ways. Books and classes on nutrition and biochemistry, which will lead you to quality foods and products are important, yet, this doesn't have to mean you are spending MORE, just differently. For example, if you take a look at Statistics

Canada, rice, dried beans, most fruit and vegetables, and even nuts, don't make the list of highest priced grocery foods. [1] The list includes meat, cheese, some processed foods, bread, and soda. Things that are not *all that* good for us are amongst the most expensive. It is statistically cheaper to live healthily; groceries, fewer medical bills, and fewer days missed at work theoretically should amount to higher energy levels, a clearer mind, and more opportunities. I also found I saved money buying quality products and supplements that actually worked, instead of buying the cheap multi-vitamin and vitamin C value packs that were hard on my stomach, so I would let them sit and expire in the cupboard... *what a waste of money.* Another thing is fad diets and "band-aid solutions." Don't even get me started. What we truly need is to educate ourselves on the human body and treat it as our forever home, providing it with the structure it needs from quality foods and products.

I have studied for years academically to understand cause and effect, reaction and deficiencies. I can keep myself comfortable fairly easy if I don't let triggers in, but I can also correct myself when something in my body hurts. I experience pains very often in different ways, but research, self study, and taking note of my day have really helped me to identify the root cause instead of just treating it symptomatically. This is part of listening to your body, getting to know your triggers.

What Sets A Person Off Balance?

The answer is: a deficiency. When we take a look at human cellular function, nutrition really is the building block. It is mind boggling that doctors are not highly versed in nutrition. Biology and biochemistry have absolutely everything to do with nutrition and the human connection to food. A human cell is made up of roughly two-thirds water, and the rest consists of macronutrients and micronutrients. Macronutrients are the ones we need in large amounts: protein, fats, carbohydrates, as well as dietary fiber and fluids, *which are the two that most people forget about.* Micronutrients are vitamins and minerals which we need small amounts of. We need adequate amounts of both macros and micros to achieve homeostasis. Homeostasis can be defined as the stable condition of an organism and of its internal environment. The stable condition is the condition of optimal functioning for the organism and is dependent on many variables, such as body temperature and fluid balance, being kept within certain pre-set limits. Other variables include the pH of extracellular fluid, the concentrations of sodium, potassium, and calcium ions, as well as that of the blood sugar level, and these need to be regulated despite changes in the environment, diet, or level of activity. [2] A medicated body is not the answer to optimal health or balance (homeostasis) - a well nourished body is.

A plant-based diet delivers micronutrients to the body as well as clean and easily digestible macronutrients. Being plant-based means that 80% of your diet, the base, is from a plant source: veggies, fruits, herbs, nuts, and grains. Since two-thirds of our body is fluid and our society commonly suffers from dehydration, it is best to have a good amount of your diet consist of items with high water content: celery, lettuce, fruits, juice, etc. There are many elements and lifestyle habits that lead to dehydration such as caffeine, alcohol, sugar, incorrect humidity levels, and lack of proper micronutrients. Additionally, stress and busy lifestyles also influence this. So what does dehydration have to do with hormones and overall health? Water is made up of hydrogen and oxygen. Proper hydration will lead to proper oxygen levels, which delivers nutrients to our cells. Increasing oxygen levels in our blood helps our cells to function properly and fight off illness and disease.

In 1931, Dr. Warburg won his first Nobel Prize for proving cancer is caused by a lack of oxygen respiration in cells. He stated in an article titled, *The Prime Cause and Prevention of Cancer*, "The cause of cancer is no longer a mystery, we know it occurs whenever any cell is denied 60% of its oxygen requirements..."

Hemoglobin is a main part of red blood cells and binds oxygen. Anemia is a condition that develops when your blood lacks enough healthy red blood cells or hemoglobin. If you have too few or abnormal red blood cells or your hemoglobin is abnormal or low, the cells in your body will not get enough oxygen. Anemia is something you can fix, without consuming meat, contrary to common belief. Anemia is caused by low iron levels and also low oxygen to the cells. Iron binds to oxygen from the air you breathe, carries it throughout your body, and releases it so it can enter your cells and tissues. It is all connected. Anemia can cause heavy bleeding, fatigue, leg cramps, insomnia, and shortness of breath. Heavy menstrual bleeding is a cause for anemia and an ongoing symptom of it. Anemic symptoms are similar to that of estrogen dominance and abnormal cellular growth in female precancers and cancer. An adequate intake of iron is needed in the body but does not have to come from meat. The required daily amount (RDA) of iron for men and postmenopausal women is 8 mg. Because of women's monthly blood losses, the RDA for premenopausal women jumps to 18 mg. The RDA during pregnancy jumps even more to 27 mg to provide adequate iron stores for the infant. Many women suffer from anemia because of a mix of things: poor diet, low vitamin C intake, chemically lined sanitary products (tampons and pads) that irritate and increase blood loss, and estrogen dominance. Anemia is extremely common. It seems if people haven't been diagnosed with it, they still feel they have it. Doctors prescribe meat and medication; why is no one talking about oxygen?

We are suffocating when we are sick.

Oxygen rich foods include lemons, avocados, berries, carrots, currants, ripe bananas, celery, garlic, dates, alfalfa sprouts, apricots, sweet apples, sweet grapes and pears, passion fruit, raisins, pineapple, vegetable juices, fruit juices, chicory, kiwis, asparagus, watercress, and seaweed.

Iron rich foods / Iron has two types: heme and non-heme. Heme iron is only present in animal flesh. Non-heme iron can be found naturally in tofu, legumes, spinach, raisins, and other plant foods. It is the form of iron used in fortified and enriched foods such as breakfast cereals, bread, and pasta. As an excess of iron is highly toxic; the human body tightly regulates the amount of iron it absorbs. Depending on the body's need for iron, we absorb approximately 15-35% of the heme iron we ingest but significantly less of the non-heme iron. Vitamin C-rich foods enhance the absorption of non-heme iron. Thus, you will absorb more iron from legumes, for example, if, when you eat them, you also eat fresh tomatoes or an orange.

Micronutrients for red blood cells are vitamin B12 and folate. I am sure these have been recommended to you if you are a woman. You may be able to boost your blood oxygen levels by adding these to your diet. Folate, also called vitamin B9, and folic acid being the synthetic version, helps your body make red blood cells — the iron-rich cells that carry oxygen in your blood. Vitamin B12 helps you make hemoglobin, which is the protein that contains oxygen-carrying iron. Boost your folate intake by including citrus fruits and dark leafy greens. You can get more vitamin B12 through nutritional yeast, fortified nut-milks, and supplementation.

Soy was mentioned in the form of tofu and nut-milks, and it will be recommended frequently throughout. So I would like to debunk the myths around soy. [3]

Soy has been a target in the media for most of my life. Even while Harvard and many other esteemed establishments were explaining the science, the media did not see it this way. There is much conspiracy about the influence the dairy industry has in the media. We were led to believe, *and many still do believe,* that soy mimics estrogen causing more estrogen to be present in the body. The problem lies in how people understand this. Mimic does not necessarily mean to duplicate and create more; it could imitate. The phytoestrogen present in soy attaches itself to estrogen but appears to neutralize it / block it. If you are estrogen dominant, *as I was*, soy may be a solution for you. Many doctors and wellness professionals, including myself, do not recommend isoflavone (a phytoestrogen found chiefly in soybeans) supplements or pills. I am not partial to taking soy products as nutritional supplementation. I prefer to consume it as a dinner protein source in a more natural form. For supplementation I gravitate towards pea protein, rice protein and quinoa protein, or blends. In any case, relying on *one thing* for our health will never work. Our bodies are made up of many vitamins and minerals, and variety is key to a well-balanced diet.

In a 2004-2009 study supported in part by Susan Komen's Breast Cancer Research Foundation, Massachusetts Department of Public Health Breast Cancer Research Program, and the United States Public Health Service RO1 AT00863, researchers evaluated breast cancer being significantly less prevalent among Asian women, whose diets contain high intake of soy products and green tea. The study suggests that dietary soy phytochemical concentrate (SPC) plus green tea (GT) may be used as a potential effective dietary regimen for inhibiting progression of estrogen-dependent breast cancer. Multiple studies have also demonstrated that components in dietary soy have anti-carcinogenic effects on breast tumors. The chemopreventive properties of the soy isoflavone genistein have been the subject of extensive *in vitro* and *in vivo* research. [4]

"Even though soy protein has little direct effect on cholesterol, soy foods are good for the heart and blood vessels because they usually replace less healthful choices, like red meat, and because they deliver plenty of polyunsaturated fat, fiber, vitamins, and minerals, and are low in saturated fat... Phytoestrogens don't always mimic estrogens. In some tissues, they actually block the action of estrogen. If soy's estrogen-blocking action occurs in the breast, then eating soy could, in theory, reduce the risk of breast cancer because estrogen stimulates the growth and multiplication of breast and breast cancer cells."

~ HARVARD

Frank Hu, a professor of nutrition and epidemiology at the Harvard School of Public Health, says that studies in Asian populations have found that diets high in soy products correlate with lower cancer rates. Studies in Western populations have been less clear, in part because fewer people consume a lot of soy. As for determining safe levels of soy consumption, Hu says, "Soy consumption has been very high historically in Asian populations, and there is no reason for them to reduce their consumption."

Livestrong recently in 2017 stated, "Soybean and related soy products are high in phytoestrogens, plant estrogens with weak activity in humans. These weaker estrogens appear to bind to the estrogen receptor on breast and ovarian cells and block the stronger human form of estrogen from binding. Overall this leads to lower levels of estrogen in the body and a reduced cancer risk."

Adding non-GMO or organic soy and tofu as a protein source into your diet a few times a week appears to have positive effects on the overall health of a human body.

What Do Deficiencies Look and Feel Like?

Deficiency means a lack of, or shortage: weakness. Vitamins and minerals at an adequate level keep us optimal, meaning best, at our best.

Ailments: digestive issues, body aches, osteoporosis, arthritis, hormonal changes and imbalances, eczema, anxiety, and menstrual cramps
• Calcium: Dairy is high in calcium; however, calcium slows down digestion. Since dairy is not balanced with magnesium which relaxes the body and digestive tract, consuming too much dairy can cause constipation. The body has two ways of detoxing: expelling, and through the skin. If we are constipated, we may experience eczema or acne and skin issues. A dairy allergy is also known to cause eczema and other skin issues such as rashes. While calcium is known to keep bones strong and prevent osteoporosis (typically as a result of hormonal changes, or deficiency of calcium or vitamin D), dairy is not a great source for this because it is extremely acidic. Acidic foods pull our reserved vitamins and minerals in the body's attempt to neutralize acidity. Too much calcium can interfere with absorption of other minerals (it is very easy to have excessive amounts of calcium from consuming dairy often) and even lead to kidney stones. Consuming dairy for health purposes, in my studied opinion, is counter intuitive. Excess fat in the diet can have an adverse effect to calcium, again making dairy not such a great option. Calcium is good for reducing menstrual cramps and is important for the secretion of hormones and enzymes, but consuming it from plant-based sources is ideal. Cheese, for example, has 750+ mg of calcium, whereas parsley and almonds both still have over 200 mg per serving. Parsley? Yes, add that to everything. Corn tortillas, pumpkin seeds, and cabbage are other great sources of calcium.
• Magnesium: Magnesium has calming properties. It is the "slow down" vitamin. It is great for digestion, inflammation, aches and pain, anxiety, and insomnia. There are different types of magnesium in the marketplace. While magnesium is calming, too much can be a bad thing - just how too much calcium isn't good. Magnesium can lead to loose stools and gastrointestinal distress. My favorite type is magnesium glycinate because it is the best-absorbed form of magnesium and one of the gentlest on the stomach.
• A balanced amount of magnesium and calcium will make for a happy stomach. Almonds, spinach, and sesame seeds are rich in both. It is recommended to have a 3:2 ratio of calcium:magnesium.

Ailments: stress, lack of interest and poor concentration (sometimes mistaken for depression or hormonal imbalances), cramps, anxiety and tension
• *Well, we are all familiar with things that cause stress, and this book dives deep into physical stress, so for now, I will only provide the remedy.* If stress is leading to alcohol or caffeine use / dependency and dehydration, you will want to take note of your B vitamin levels.
• Vitamin B5 helps to produce anti-stress hormones known as DHEA / steroids. It works with other B vitamins and is often why we see a combination of B vitamins in one supplement. Folate aids in its absorption. Some foods which contain vitamin B5 and can be incorporated into your diet are lentils, mushrooms, avocados, and broccoli.

The simple solution over remembering all of this, is to eat plant-based.

Ailments: PMS, menopause, depression, lack of hormone production, water retention, anxiety, irritability, cramps, lack of energy, poor diet (processed and refined foods), alcohol and smoking, birth control pill, use infrequent dream recall
• Vitamin B6 is another great "happy hormones" vitamin that you will also find in lentils and broccoli. Wheat germ has high levels of vitamin B6, and you will find it in bananas and some presence of it in many vegetables. Combine it with other B vitamins, as well as magnesium and zinc.

Ailments: frequent cold, weak immune system, stress, pollutants (in air, smoking, alcohol, fried foods), pimples
• Vitamin C is known to loosen bowels. Consuming too much of it can be uncomfortable, and you don't want to end up dehydrated. Oranges are a great source of vitamin C, but some foods that are even higher are peppers, cabbage, watercress (actually contains most of these above vitamins), cauliflower, and strawberries. Grapefruits aren't quite as high as oranges, but are also a very good source and are more alkaline forming in the body - same with lemons!

Ailments: acne / hormonal acne / greasy skin, low fertility, frequent depression, lack of appetite, and pale skin (generally looking and feeling crummy)
• Zinc: I think it is important to dive into zinc as we did with calcium. It is not often referenced in relation to hormones as much as the B vitamins are, but zinc actually controls hormones which are messengers from reproductive organs (testes and ovaries) and aids in the ability to cope with stress. Zinc promotes a healthy nervous system and brain. Zinc is a component of over 200 enzymes in the body and is essential for growth while important for healing.

• When balanced with copper, gastrointestinal irritation, anaemia, and depraved appetite will be controlled. It is possible to have too much zinc, so in my opinion, it is best to get it from food sources instead of supplementing, but there are gentle and safe supplements as well. Copper assists with the transport of iron. Rich sources of copper include legumes, nuts, and seeds. They all work together in harmony. Unfortunately, with the way our food is cultivated these days, zinc is not as present as it should be. Oysters are said to be an aphrodisiac, and I think that is because they are extremely high in zinc which works as a messenger for hormones to and from reproductive organs. For plant-based sources, try ginger root, pecans, split and green peas, Brazil nuts, peanuts, and, again, almonds.

Too much calcium isn't great for zinc absorption. You will also need to be consuming protein, so the nut and pea options are great sources. Sugar and alcohol will have adverse effects as well as bread. If you feel you have a zinc deficiency, avoid those three things.

Ailments: joint pain, muscle twitches, cramping
• Manganese: Although not directly related to hormones, it is important for insulin production and essential for reproduction of red blood cell synthesis. It plays an important role with enzymes and general overall health. Pineapple, blackberries, and raspberries are the foods for this! If you are drawn to these foods often, your body might be looking for manganese. Manganese is sometimes promoted to reduce cramps and is also found in endive, known as the women's leaf.

Ailments: weight gain, slow digestion, bloating, constipation, cough, sinus problems, osteoarthritis, fat gain at waist line
• Bromelain is an enzyme found in pineapple juice and in the pineapple stem. WebMD says, "People use it as a medicine." Bromelain is used for reducing swelling (inflammation), especially of the nose and sinuses, after surgery or injury. It is also used for hay fever, treating a bowel condition that includes swelling and ulcers (ulcerative colitis), removing dead and damaged tissue after a burn (debridement), preventing the collection of water in the lung (pulmonary edema), relaxing muscles, stimulating muscle contractions, slowing clotting, improving the absorption of antibiotics, preventing cancer, shortening labor, and helping the body get rid of fat. It is also used for preventing muscle soreness after intense exercise. This use has been studied, and the evidence suggests synthetic bromelain doesn't work for this. It is best found in FRESH pineapple.

Slice up some fresh pineapple!

Ailments: poor sleep, insulin resistance, imbalanced hormones, depression, inflammation, blood clotting, eczema, PMS or breast pain, water retention
• Omega 3 (ALA, EPA, DHA): There is not a wealth of sources for this. It is in fish and flax seeds, as well as walnuts, chia seeds, and shelled hemp seeds. Algae, egg yolk, and sunflower seeds are some other options. Flax, chia and / or hemp seeds go a long way. They can be blended into pasta sauce or smoothies, topped on salads, and made into baked goods such as bread and treats, even gluten-free ones! In vegan dishes, they work as a binding agent as a replacement for eggs; so if you are going plant-based, you can still get your omegas.
All of the aforementioned vitamins promote absorption of Omega 3.

Other "happy hormone" vitamins are minerals are:
• Selenium for thyroid is found in Brazil nuts and mushrooms; this may be a good one to supplement as the whole food sources are limited.
• Iodine for thyroid deficiencies can commonly be found in potatoes, iodized salt, and legumes, and can also be absorbed through the skin.

The simple solution over remembering all of this, is to eat plant-based. At least 80% of your diet should be plant-based. Eat a diet rich in a variety of nuts, seeds, beans, and legumes (lentils and peas) which provide important micronutrients as well as good protein and fats. Brazil nuts and peas come up frequently for "happy hormone" foods. Brazil nuts are a bit pricey, but peas are cheap! Balance out your consumption and budget to get a wide variety of foods.

Add hearty vegetables such as cauliflower, spinach, and broccoli, and try out new things like watercress on top of salads. Pineapple is amazing in so many ways, especially for digestion, reducing belly fat, breaking down food, and delivering manganese. I add pineapple to pasta and pizza as well as a grilled pineapple on veggie burgers. Snacking on a variety of nuts, seeds, and fruit, even just once a day, will drastically improve your well being.

My favorite things to commonly eat that are also super healthy are...

- Almonds
- Fresh lemons (for salad dressing and in water)
- Avocados
- Spinach (on top of toast, cooked in pasta, in a smoothie, salad, etc., - in everything)
- Pineapple
- Parsley (sandwich, salad, stir-fry, pizza, pasta, rice dishes, potato dishes)
- Cauliflower (cauliflower wings, pizza base, mashed, ROASTED in the oven is so easy with pepper, paprika, garlic and onion salt)
- Spirulina and chlorophyll / chlorella (these keep me so healthy and can be taken via supplement or added into smoothies, baking, etc. See chapter 1 for more information)
- Fiber: Majority of people do not get adequate amounts of soluble and insoluble fiber, and a lack of fiber can lead to IBS, gastrointestinal issues, irregular bowel movements, hemorrhoids, affect ulcerative colitis, a reduction in vitamin and mineral absorption, and dehydration. Fiber is important. Do some research into it, and we really could *and will* write an entire book on the subject.

If you have a health condition you would like to correct but are a picky eater or have food allergies or preferences, I suggest doing some research into your condition, finding out what kind of deficiencies cause it, then researching what foods are high in that vitamin or mineral. The options are plentiful. Nutritionists have a wide variety of education. You may find some instruct differently than others, so feel free to reach out to them and ask some questions first on what kind of diets they recommend. Just because someone has a health title or degree and tells you to eat meat, or go paleo, or go vegan, or go on medication, does not mean they are right. A nutritional and lifestyle assessment should be done, packed with education on the "why and how" of foods. I always recommend asking a wide variety of people for help but also doing your due diligence. Read some basic chemistry books as well as food science books.

There are only so many vitamins and minerals, and once you get to know what your body gravitates towards and what it needs more of, you can add the right foods and supplements into your diet.

Do We Actually Need Supplements?

Through out my studies, it was taught as a general rule of thumb that women eating 1600 calories or fewer per day, and men consuming 1800 calories or less per day, will not be able to meet their nutritional requirements simply because there is not enough food being consumed. While at the same time, both di Bonaventura and Dr. Delichatsios say that a woman *can* meet her nutrient needs through food alone, even if she eats 1,500 calories (or less) per day. "It's not an issue of food quantity but rather food quality. Even a low-calorie diet can have the needed vitamins and minerals," says Dr. Delichatsios. The only exception is vitamin D. There are mixed results. Let's look at this closer.

Eatthismuch.com is a good resource for meal planning to stay within a calorie range and also meet your macronutrient requirements. Unfortunately, at the time of this book, it does not address micronutrients, and as we have learned, some people may have conditions, low absorption issues, or lifestyle habits that will require them to take more of a specific vitamin or mineral. If we look at a 1600 calorie vegetarian meal, it has a wide range of colors (different colored vegetables and fruits tend to be good for different things, see chapter 17). Looking at the average meal plan on the website though, it is very hard for me to imagine many people are having a protein shake for breakfast, salad and celery sticks topped with peanut butter for lunch, and ending their day with 2 oz pasta with veggies and a side of edamame. People are more than likely having bread for breakfast and / or lunch with cheese, butter, and some sort of processed meat, with a few healthy shakes or salad per week, but not every day, and a dinner serving of pasta, potatoes, or rice usually outweighing the veggies on the plate. We are far from balanced as a society. As mentioned, this website at this time does not factor-in micronutrients. So how do we need to eat to get all our micros on 1600 calories? Here is a meal plan posted from Harvard Health. [5]

Harvard Health 1,200-calorie sample menu that meets the daily DRIs*
for a woman 51 to 70 years of age

Breakfast	Lunch
8oz nonfat yogurt	1 small whole-wheat pita
½ cup sliced papaya	Green salad:
½ cup sliced kiwi	*1 cup dark green lettuce*
1oz (14 halves) walnuts	1 red or orange pepper
4oz skim milk	1 cup grape tomatoes
	½ cup edamame beans
	1 tablespoon unsalted sunflower seeds.
	Salad dressing made with 1 tablespoon olive oil, bal-samic vinegar, and pepper

Dinner

4oz broiled wild salmon and yogurt sauce (1 tablespoon Greek-style nonfat yogurt, 1 teaspoon. lemon juice, 1 clove chopped garlic)

¼ cup cooked barley and ¼ cup cooked lentils with spices to taste

1 cup steamed baby bok choy

Dietary reference intakes.

Menu provides 1,155 calories:

33% of calories from fat, 40% from carbohydrate, and 27% from protein

Vitamins and minerals and their amounts in the sample menu, above
(DRIs are listed in *Dietary reference intakes)

Vitamin A, 1,031 mcg (700 mcg)	Vitamin B12, 10.6 mcg (2.4 mcg)
Vitamin C, 383 mg (75 mg)	Pantothenic acid, 5.5 mg (5 mg)
Vitamin D, 12 mcg (10 mcg)	Calcium, 1,222 mg (1,200 mg)
Vitamin E, 11 mg (15 mg)	Copper, 900 mcg (1,156 mcg)
Vitamin K, 156 mcg (90 mcg)	Iron, 11 mg (8 mg)
Thiamin, 1.3 mg (1.1 mg)	Magnesium, 355 mg (320 mg)
Riboflavin, 1.8 mg (1.1 mg)	Manganese, 2.8 mg (1.8 mg)
Niacin, 14 mg (14 mg)	Phosphorus, 1,530 mg (700 mg)
Vitamin B6, 2.23 mg (1.5 mg)	Selenium, 90 mcg (55 mcg)
Folate, 556 mcg (400 mcg)	Zinc, 8.6 mg (8 mg)
Potassium, 4.7 g (4.7 g)	

Note: Biotin, choline, and chromium are not precisely measured in foods and thus not included in our analysis.
Source: Ellen di Bonaventura, R.D., clinical dietitian, Massachusetts General Hospital, Boston, MA.

Hmm, looking at this, my first comment is how many people eat papaya, not to mention papaya, kiwi, bok choy, walnuts and edamame, all in the same day? As soon as we replace one fruit for another fruit, or one vegetable for another vegetable, we change the nutritional make of the day. Second, a lot of people do not eat fish or dairy and may have intolerances to a few things on this meal plan. I DO feel that we need to add supplements within our daily food intake. Our food is also not cultivated the way it used to be. There are countless studies proving that our produce now, compared to the 1970s, is 14% to 37% less nutrient dense. A landmark study on the topic by Donald Davis and his team of researchers from the University of Texas at Austin's Department of Chemistry and Biochemistry was published in December 2004 in the Journal of the American College of Nutrition. They studied U.S. Department of Agriculture nutritional data from both 1950 and 1999 for 43 different vegetables and fruits, finding "reliable declines" in the amount of protein, calcium, phosphorus, iron, riboflavin (vitamin B2), and vitamin C over the past half century. Davis and his colleagues chalk up this declining nutritional content to the preponderance of agricultural practices designed to improve traits (size, growth rate, pest resistance: pesticides and GMOs) other than nutrition. [6,7,8,9]

Natural, organic, plant-based, and nutrient dense foods solve a lot of problems for our earth and our body. It is what we are connected to. If connecting the dots, eating plant-based can improve stressors around physical and mental health, relationships, success, comfortability, financials, happiness, the earth's environment, and respiratory health and can aid in creating happy, prosperous, more responsible, and kinder people. We can embody stress, or we can embody compassion. A nurtured body leads to nurtured heath which creates a nurtured earth, and vice versa. It is all connected.

Further reading on micronutrients and cellular health
www.hindawi.com/journals/bmri/2013/597282/
Nutritional composition decline of fruits and vegetables
http://hortsci.ashspublications.org/content/44/1/15.full

THANK YOU

To Josh Rudner for sharing an article that helped start my journey; it was an article about how ALL disease starts at a cellular level. Natalie Cadieux, you came into my life and helped me make a three month impactful change. Although I am not a consultant anymore, thank you Arbonne and all the consultants I met. You are my best friends, and helped me discover a better life for myself. Thank you to the coauthors for joining this book, trusting me to guide it, and sharing your story. We are allowing people to follow in our sustainable footprint.
~ Ky-Lee Hanson

MINDFULNESS ON HER PLATE

Featuring

Effie Mitskopoulos

Jy Nanda

Charleyne Oulton

Kelly Spencer

A LIBERATING CHOICE: MINDFUL EATING

MINDFULNESS GIVES YOU CHOICE IN HOW TO NOURISH YOUR BODY, MIND, AND HEART.

by Effie Mitskopoulos

Honours Bachelor of Science in Biology and Psychology, (Hons)B.Sc.,
Masters of Social Work, MSW
Registered Social Worker, RSW
Certified Hypnotherapist, C.Hyp.
Certified Yoga Teacher, CYT
Certified Kundalini Yoga Teacher, C-KYT
Reiki Master

Effie Mitskopoulos

Effie Mitskopoulos, founder of Soul Body Healer, is a registered social worker specializing in holistic psychotherapy. She combines customized Western interventions with hypnosis, mindfulness, yoga, and energy work. Her commitment to helping others stems from her own healing journey. Despite hardships in her life, she kept receiving messages that there was more to life than suffering and kept pushing on. Many times she felt like giving up, but hope and persistence kept her seeking knowledge, authenticity, spirituality, and ultimately, wellness. Her journey was catapulted in 2010 by practicing Kundalini yoga and becoming a yoga teacher. She came to realize that healing occurs on all levels: mind, body, and soul. Because much discomfort stems from a mental-emotional-energetic cause, practicing mindfulness and hypnosis shifts unconscious programs, thus aiding in managing emotional states, while Reiki and yoga bring balance and strength to the body and energetic systems by releasing unresolved emotions and energy blockages.

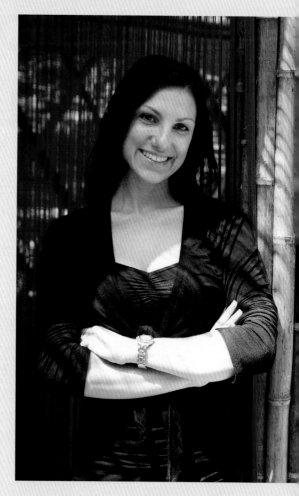

Effie has provided programs for thousands of people in many populations ranging from stress management, depression, anxiety, chronic pain, addiction, and trauma. She believes that every individual has special gifts and has the strength to heal themselves. It is her passion to help her clients uncover the root cause of their discomfort and release distressing patterns so they live happy, peaceful, and meaningful lives. Her vision is the upliftment of humanity - for people to feel whole, well, and free to express themselves fully so that every interaction is loving and compassionate, supporting a peaceful world.

WWW.SOULBODYHEALER.COM
e: soulbodyhealer@gmail.com | fb: soulbodyhealer

At any given moment, whether you're in the car, doing a task, or eating a meal, do you ever find your mind wandering? Maybe it's planning a list of tasks to complete later or worrying about a future that may never happen. It may be thinking about a past event - be it pleasant or unpleasant. When I ask my clients to journal where their attention is during a mundane task, they tend to find their minds wandering more than 50% of the time. Some neuroscientists postulate that we are only consciously aware of the present moment 5% the time! [1] How much time does *your* mind spend in the present moment where your body is? The present moment is the only place we are and can fully be. Here is the only place we can laugh, communicate, solve problems, and eat, among other things.

This mindlessness can trickle into how we choose to nourish ourselves with food. I've been practicing mindfulness for almost eight years now and seem to have a conscious grasp on my thoughts in everyday life; however, I am definitely distracted when I eat. This is something I've brought more attention to and am working on now. At mealtime, I tend to watch television, read, or engage in conversation. Where does your mind wander to when you eat? What are you "doing" at mealtime? Sometimes we may barely even taste our food! Intriguingly, studies have shown that when our mind is focused on things other than eating, digestion decreases by 30-40%. [2] Poor digestion can be felt in many ways, such as bloating, belching, diarrhea and / or constipation. When the mind is paying attention to what the body is doing in the present, the nervous system is relaxed, and optimal digestion occurs. When the nervous system detects a threat (something stressful), the fight or flight system is activated. A stress hormone called cortisol causes many biochemical changes, one of which is blood flowing out of our digestive system and into our muscles so that we can "get out of danger." In this state, digestion slows or even stops, which is when you feel all those unpleasant symptoms, not just physically but also mentally. For me, bloating and belching not only made me physically uncomfortable, but also triggered thoughts of feeling fat which was not supportive of feeling good about myself. The stress response can be triggered just by our thoughts alone. So, if we are thinking / watching / reading something even mildly stressful, the body turns on this response. A wandering mind doesn't just affect how we digest food, but also influences the foods we choose and the quantity and frequency we eat. This impacts our body's functioning and how we feel in and about our body.

When we are not paying attention to the present moment, unconscious beliefs influence our thoughts and emotions, which in turn trigger certain behaviour. For example, growing up, every family had norms regarding how and what they ate, and we learn these associations actively of course, but as we grow up, these associations are so ingrained in us on a subliminal level, it influences our eating habits, choices, and patterns. Perhaps we learned that we "mustn't be wasteful," or "ungrateful," or "must eat everything on the plate," and, hence today, we lick our plates clean even if we are full. We may have learned to temporarily avoid uncomfortable emotions and create a pleasurable one by eating sugary or fatty foods (e.g. eating ice cream on a bad day). For others, eating may not be as important and is done quickly to "get the job done and to go onto more important things." There are many beliefs and behaviours which influence our well-being. Being mindful is a non-judgmental observation of your internal and external experience. You are able to explore why and how you eat, uncover the unconscious habits and beliefs, and choose which ones to keep, discard, or replace. Doing so gives you the power to choose to optimize your body's functioning, self-esteem, and overall health and wellness. Mindfulness not only creates relaxation for optimal digestion but also gives you a choice in how to nourish the body, mind, and heart.

Mindful Eating Is A Form Of Mindfulness

Mindfulness has been practiced for thousands of years. It involves focusing on the present moment in a neutral way, approaching each moment with a particular mindset, with curiosity, trust, patience, and acceptance of the present experience. There is no goal or purpose. It is practiced solely for its sake, and we let go of any desired outcome. [3] This is quite a foreign concept since our minds like to be in "doing mode," and we've learned in the past to categorize and judge our experiences. That's why it's called a practice. As we apply this perspective to our experiences, magical things begin to happen. Many studies have shown that just eight weeks of a mindfulness program produces greater feelings of happiness, lowered pain, reduced anxiety and depression, better sleep patterns, increased compassion, and a greater ability to stay calm. [4] In this state, we cultivate a calmer response to the world that is in line with our goals instead of a stressful reaction. For instance, I may come home after a stressful day at work and have the urge to eat cookies instead of dinner. I am mindful and understand without judgment that ultimately, that would leave my mind, body, and heart unsatisfied. So, I choose to eat a healthy dinner and eat one cookie. Mindful eating helps us learn how to intuitively nourish our bodies without overeating or undereating and choose foods that make us feel happy and vital. After all, food is meant to fuel this beautiful temple of ours! We pay attention with all senses to the physical and emotional sensations of the entire eating process. We gain a reciprocal relationship with our bodies when we communicate about hunger and satisfaction.

> "Mindful eating replaces self-criticism with self nurturing. It replaces shame with your own self wisdom."
> ~ DR. JAN CHOZEN BAYS

Discovery: Food And Mood

As we bring awareness to the whole process of choosing how to nourish ourselves, we may find that certain foods and food practices cause discomfort in the body and / or mind. We are able to investigate food sensitivities and explore the foods that make us feel well or unwell. We may find that certain foods help us feel more energetic and happy while others make us feel sluggish and icky. For instance, I know when I eat fresh salads and vegetables, I feel light, energetic, and confident in my body. Conversely, when I eat chips, my head feels heavy and starts to ache, and I feel nauseous, which in turn triggers judgmental thoughts about my body and the behaviour of eating the chips in the first place. We may also notice how our emotional states affect our food choices. For instance, stress releases cortisol, which causes us to crave foods like sugar, fat, and salt for quick energy. Choosing these types of foods ultimately causes our bodies to feel tired, unhealthy, and heavy. [5] Research also shows that we may choose to eat to escape (the awareness of) a stressful state, [6] and neurologically, it temporarily does help us escape. Ingesting sugar improves mood by activating the dopamine and opioid receptors, which are linked to pain relief and pleasure. [7] Furthermore, sugar is the dominant form of energy our body needs for its processes. Thus, this pleasure pathway is activated for our survival, so we continue to reward ourselves with this life-giving substance. However, the problem is a lot of sugar is refined nowadays, and all the good nutrients and fiber have been removed. Thus, this reward comes at a high cost - excess weight, diabetes, sluggishness, headaches, etc.

> "We learn who is hungry (the body or the mind?) and for what, then respond by nourishing it in the best way possible!"
>
> ~ J.C. BAYS

Also affecting our mood is the food practice of not eating regularly or leaving too much space between meals. Our blood sugar drops, and this can cause feelings of irritability, depression, and fatigue. There's a biological urge to find something to eat so we can boost our mood and blood sugar levels, and the easiest thing is to eat something high in sugar. Here, we are operating from a "mindless" state and choose foods we have learned from prior experience that do the job quickly. We may have learned that by eating a chocolate bar, we temporarily fill that need, but then our energy crashes (as does our mood) when the energy from the sugar gets used up. And we are back to where we first started or often worse. The key is to first not get to that point of starvation so that our biological urges don't overrun our conscious choice of what and how to eat. It's a lot easier to mindfully choose an item to eat when our body is not screaming at us. Secondly, it is helpful to choose foods that release energy slowly to avoid crashes like whole fruits and vegetables, lean protein, whole grains, oats, and good fats like nuts and seeds.

Food can even be used as a substance, like drugs or alcohol, to soothe one's emotions, create states that are more desirable than the present one, and avoid what's really going on inside. By tuning into my thoughts, emotions, and sensations, I learned a lot about why I use certain foods like sugar, chocolate, and coffee for reasons other than nourishing my body. I wasn't aware of my sugar addiction. Sometimes, I would eat spoonfuls of honey to meet the need. Did my body actually want honey for nourishment? Probably not. Being mindful of the cravings, I learned (and am continuously learning) that sometimes these cravings were born out of feeling overwhelmed, where there were too many tasks on my plate, other times boredom, loneliness, or just to taste something good and create pleasure. Furthermore, I learned how sensitive I was to sugar during a twelve-day elimination cleanse. Not eating sugar caused me to feel irritable and snappy, and I was even dreaming of honey! At the end, I was supposed to slowly reintroduce the eliminated foods back into my diet, sugar being last. But at my niece's fourth birthday party, how could I deny her sweet little face offering me some ice cream cake? That night I found myself lying on the couch with a severe headache, like a jackhammer was burrowing into my brain. I was nauseated, and my mind spinning out of control. I was drunk on sugar! The next morning I had a sugar hangover! Today, I consciously watch how many grams I take in and choose healthier sugar sources. However, I have yet to cut it out completely and do not judge myself for having some.

During a tour of my new apartment, my friends found my chocolate cupboard. I've become aware of it as my security blanket for connection, comfort, love, and pleasure. Sometimes I eat chocolate every day; sometimes I go weeks without. It all depends on my mood! Those times I have a heavy client load and forget to bring dark chocolate to work, I really feel its absence. A tape of the following thoughts plays in my mind: *Oh no, I wish I brought it, maybe I should buy some during lunch? No, you have a big stash at home...* how silly? No, no judgment here. The thoughts are just thoughts. I choose to focus on my clients and administrative work, and the chocolate urge eventually passes. This is another way of using mindfulness to overcome cravings, not just for exploration, but as a tool to choose behaviors that are best in line with my values and virtues.

Coffee, however, is another story. About seven years ago, I experienced adrenal fatigue. My adrenal glands were overworked pumping out cortisol from prolonged stress that they and I began feeling very tired, no matter how much sleep I got. In this state, it is advised to relax and not work the adrenal glands if they don't need to be. So, I stopped drinking coffee for two years. I know it might sound impossible, but it can be done! Since I started reintroducing it back into my life, I realized what I use it for. I observe myself planning my consumption as a "reward" for a hard day's work or to focus when I have a lot that needs to be done. Essentially,

I feel more pleasure doing all the work if I'm sipping on coffee. I also notice I have thoughts such as, *Life is exciting, and it is worth living.* It is as though the beautiful coffee bean is whispering sweet hymns in my ear! The key is to be aware of all that you are feeling and experiencing in the moment, so it's a conscious choice. I choose coffee in this moment and am aware of the consequences - comfortable and uncomfortable. I hope my personal accounts have given you examples to relate to or inspiration to observe and discover your experiences with food!

How To Eat Mindfully

Mindful eating begins even before we eat. Consider how hungry you are. What are you craving? What do your taste buds say they want? Is this based on an emotional urge or an urge to fuel yourself? What food will make you feel energized instead of slow, bloated, heavy, or hyper?

Mindfulness practitioners typically teach the following exercise with a raisin because of its distinct appearance, smell, taste, and possible associations, but you can choose any food. Observe the entire experience with openness, curiosity, patience, and non-judgment.

1. Choose the food and appreciate where it came from. Appreciate the people who tended to the soil, grew it, and picked it, all the processes that led it to be so beautifully standing in front of you.

2. Place it in your hand (or on your fork / spoon). Appreciate the food's outward appearance. What does it look like (color, texture)? Squish it between your fingers. Observe any sound. Are there any associations that pop into your mind? Thoughts? Emotions? Likes? Dislikes?

3. Bring the food close to your nose. What does it smell like? Can you distinguish more than one flavor? Do you begin to salivate? Note any mental and emotional associations.

4. Place the food (or take a small bite) in your mouth without chewing. Notice its texture and temperature. Rediscover all the unique flavours of the food. Notice the urge to chew and apply curiosity, without necessarily needing to follow the urge and chew.

5. Begin to chew the food, at least twenty slow bites. Does the taste change? Notice what's happening in your body and mind. Notice the urge to swallow, but resist it. Enjoy the act of chewing - the feel of your teeth and jaw muscles working. Digestion starts in the mouth. The teeth break up the food into smaller pieces, and saliva has an enzyme that chemically breaks down carbohydrates.

6. Swallow. Follow the sensation of the food moving down your esophagus. Tune into peristalsis - the automatic contraction of the esophagus that moves food to the stomach for further digestion.

7. Tune in to the wisdom of your body. It knows how to break down food into molecules that are then used to heal, nourish, and revitalize itself.

Get to know all your automatic reactions, urges, and consequences to the food you eat. What is truly nourishing your body, and what is an urge that fills other needs? Use these next five principles when mindfully eating to bring more awareness to everything involved with eating. They help us listen to internal cues (hunger and satiety) and use external cues (slower eating, reducing portion sizes and distractions) so that we eat consciously.

Hunger Cues

Internal cues help assess whether you are eating due to actual hunger or if you're reacting to an emotion (whether it be something comfortable such as eating cake to celebrate your birthday or something uncomfortable such as stress eating). The following scale has been developed to assess hunger cues so you can start and stop eating in response to what your body needs for fuel. [8] Researchers advise to begin eating no later than when your "stomach feels empty, strong desire to eat" (see #3 on the below scale) and to stop no later than "completely satisfied" (see #6 on the below scale).

Scale	Body and Mind Sensations
1	Beyond hungry, weak, light headed, headache
2	Feel sick, little energy, irritable, very hungry
3	Stomach feels empty, strong desire to eat
4	Start to think about food, feel a little hungry
5	Just starting to feel satisfied, body has enough fuel
6	Completely satisfied
7	Beyond point of satisfaction, don't need anymore food for fuel. Body says "no" but mind says "yes" to a few more bites
8	Have eaten too much, starting to feel uncomfortable
9	Feeling really uncomfortable, starting to feel sluggish
10	Beyond full, feel pain, don't want to move or even look at food

The following food journal is helpful in discovering the relation between the foods you eat and your mood (Find hunger scale in section "Hunger Cues.) [8]

Time	What I ate	Hunger Scale (1-10) before and after eating	What was I doing?	Thoughts	Emotions

Distractions

With so many distractions and things to do, it's no wonder this is the hardest principle for me to follow! Can you relate? This principle teaches us to focus on enjoying our food, without watching television, music blaring, reading, or even being on the computer. Consequently, a study showed that watching television increased intake of high-fat foods and meal frequency. Indeed, it is harder to assess how full we are (internal cues) when distracted, which leads to overeating. [9] Furthermore, we even perceive the taste of food differently when our attention is somewhere else. A study found that people perceived food to be less salty, sweet, and sour while doing a task that required a lot of attention and therefore ate more to compensate for taste. Thus, the more attention diverted away from eating, the less tasty your food is, and the more you eat! [10]

Portion Size

In order to not overeat, you can use the external cue of using smaller dishes, without refilling to automatically serve yourself smaller portions. Also, pay attention to the internal cue of how full you actually feel. People consume more when plates are bigger, if they are offered more food, or in an "all you can eat" environment. A study showed that people used the visual cue of how much was left on the plate to determine fullness instead of how full their stomachs felt. Consequently, they did not realize they had eaten up to 73% more in this environment. [11] It can be confusing to estimate proper portions. There could be a correlation between obesity rates increasing with the rise in portion sizes at restaurants, vending machines, and grocery stores. In fact, Canadian obesity rates have tripled in the last thirty years. [12,13] We don't actually need to eat all the food served to us. To get a better idea of portion sizes, Diabetes Canada suggests using your hand as a guide: one fist for fruits, grains, and starches, two hands for vegetables, your palm with the thickness of your little finger for protein, and the tip of your thumb for fat. [14] Of course, everyone has individual requirements, so tailor your intake needs to what feels best in your body.

Slower Eating Rate

Take smaller bites. Chew each bite 20 times, and pause or sip water between bites to slow down your eating rate. It takes 20 minutes for your brain to register that your body is full, hence, slowing down allows one to reduce the intake of food. [15]

Savor Food

Create a pleasurable experience for yourself with what and where you eat. Use your five senses to choose foods that are pleasing. Choose foods that are not only vibrant in color but are also pleasing in texture, taste, and smell, and nourish your body. Fixing your table and surroundings as though you were eating at a "gourmet" restaurant has also been shown to increase the taste and overall experience of eating. [15]

Paying attention to the entire eating experience helps us discover what is driving us to eat in the first place. Is it because you really need to fuel yourself, or are there unconscious beliefs and habits at play? Are you feeding your emotions or your body? When mindlessly doing tasks, unhealthy patterns are more likely to surface. Taking the time to slow down and be conscious of eating allows us to make a wise choice instead of a quick reaction. Mindful eating is also used to treat problem eating behaviours, achieve healthy weight, and cultivate a positive attitude toward eating. [15] Suspending judgment and tuning into the internal and external cues surrounding food and food environments gives us the power to intentionally create a nourishing, pleasurable, and relaxing experience for ourselves. We are able to fuel our body without overeating or undereating and create conscious eating habits so that we nourish the body, mind, and heart. My hope is that you have been inspired to discover your automatic reactions connected to eating so that you liberate the choice to nourish a happier and healthier you!

THANK YOU

I am so grateful Spirit placed all the supportive people in my path so this chapter could be manifested!

~ *Effie Mitskopoulos*

HOW TO KNOW WHEN YOU'RE OVER IT: FED UP!

TO CREATE A FULFILLING LIFE,
WE NEED TO LOOK WITHIN. THAT IS THE ONLY WAY
WE STOP FILLING THE VOID WITH FOOD.

by Jy Nanda

Fitness Instructor, F.I.T.

Jy Nanda

Jy Nanda is the founder of her own coaching business called Find Your EDGE (Education Determination Goals Experience). She is a certified coach, motivational speaker, personal trainer in-training, TEDx coach, private mentor, Dale Carnegie graduate, and advanced toastmaster, with fifteen years of retail management experience. She also holds a bachelor's in political science and government as well as a certificate in public relations. Jy is passionate about public speaking and communications, as she spends much of her time delivering workshops to help people further develop their confidence. To her, it is better to be well rounded and indispensable with knowledge so she can adapt to everyday life situations with style.

e: jynanda@hotmail.com
ig: jy_nation | fb: jy.nanda

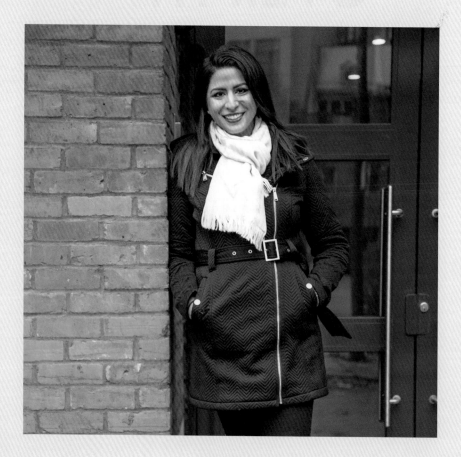

Have you ever decided you were just over it all? Done overeating, done being over exhausted, done being overstressed or even overdoing? Have you ever decided that you were done trying? Ever decided that you were fed up? This is the moment your life truly begins.

I used to be this person. I remember waking up each day, feeling drained and even more exhausted than the day before. I would dread the thought of the day ahead: waking up, showering, getting dressed, going to work, working late, eating, watching Netflix, then heading to bed. It was like a never-ending cycle. Then, I'd wake up the next day and start the cycle all over again. I was living on autopilot, and I didn't know how to stop. I felt numb. I mean really, what value did I have? I felt like a cog in a wheel, disparagingly playing my role in a machine as if I were programmed to be this way. Would I ever change?

I was and am an avid lover of personal development; there was no one I knew that loved personal development more than I did. I was obsessed with changing my mindset and loved discovering new theories, concepts, and challenges that could possibly alter my life for the better. I searched for any quick fix that could resolve the boredom I felt in my everyday life. I just felt like I wasn't experiencing life. However, no matter how much I tried to get out, I would simply find myself being pulled back in. I waited for the eureka moment to come, *that* feeling that would make all of this go away, the idea that there was something or even someone out there that could fix me or my thoughts. But here's the truth: That moment never came. I was thirty-three-years-old, 5'9 tall, weighing 222 lbs and had been on the same trajectory for most of my life. That's when it hit me. This was who I'd become. There was no magic pill; there was no ultimate truth. There was just me and my perception of the world and how I was viewing it. So what could I do now?

I first began with realizing that I was not aware of the consequences of my actions; I was living my version of a robotic trance. The first step to understanding myself was to become self-aware, and this was definitely not easy. I started by noticing my thoughts, words, and actions. The funny thing was I couldn't believe what I was thinking, saying, or doing. It was not congruent at all with what I wanted for myself.

My second step was to analyze my thoughts, feelings, and actions. This was not much easier than noticing them. Every time I would think, feel, or do something, a sense of worthlessness would wash over me. The worst part is I'd believe every mean, uncompassionate, and cruel idea that passed through my mind. It felt like I was stuck in a terrible movie I couldn't stop watching. So how could I turn it off? I realized this would not be an easy process, and I'd have to start by understanding why I thought, felt, and acted the way I did. What was my reward for continuing to be this way? Obviously, it served some kind of purpose; otherwise, I would have stopped doing it. Right?

I came to the understanding that being distracted and overdoing things did serve a purpose. It all came back to my excuses, my sense of priorities, and my daily rituals. I did not want to be seen for who I was, so I kept busy. I thought if I was always doing something, my life would have value, and people would consider me important. Ouch... I did not like admitting that at all. If I stopped doing all that I was doing, who would I be? Would I be enough? Would I be lovable? Would I be worth anything? The scariest part of all this was that I'd have to stop to find out.

I did what scared me the most. I started saying no. I started taking time off. I started to slow down. I didn't know what would come of this, but I knew that I had to take the time to find out. It wasn't easy. If anything, I was uncomfortable all the time. Saying no meant that I was rejecting others' requests. Taking time off meant feeling guilty that I couldn't get "everything" done. To me, slowing down felt like I was being lazy. None of these things felt good to me, so why was I doing them?

I did this to see myself for who I am, see what my potential was. I realized I used to say yes because I didn't want to feel guilty. For me, keeping busy meant others perceived I was doing important things. Being efficient meant I was producing value in the world. Yet, despite these reasons, nothing I said, thought, or did felt good as it wasn't meant for me. It was for others to perceive me the way I wanted to be seen, for them to see my inherent value through the work I produced. I NEVER FELT LIKE I WAS ENOUGH. So, it all made sense. I overdid everything because I felt it was never enough. The only way I found solace was through eating. Eating helped with avoiding reality. I was always hungry. It was merely a distraction, a safe place.

This is where the real work began. It meant I had to explore my life by tuning into myself and tuning out the noise of others. I created life hacks to make space in my life for myself. During this process, I released the weight I'd put on over the years, but for the first time in my life, I let go of the weight for good! I began with decluttering. Sometimes to get more out of life, you need to get rid of the excess that doesn't serve you. This could be your closet, your desk, your home. For me, this was creating space in my physical environment where I spent most of my time. I'd avoided this for many years as it is not fun at all for me. I looked at this mountain of clothes and considered this mess to be a symbol and memory of who I was, but it wasn't. It was simply a physical representation of my mental state. I believed I had an attachment to it, but it was time to let that mental mess go!

Once I began this process, I also decided to keep a gratitude journal where I recorded five things I felt grateful for in the morning and five things I felt grateful for at night. This created a

It meant I had to explore my life by tuning into myself and tuning out the noise of others.

space for seeing the abundance that was already ever-present in my life! I became less self-deprecating once I stopped focusing on what I did not have, and instead, started focusing on what I had already created in my life.

Next, I created the space to get physically active. That meant going to the gym, even when I didn't feel like it, even after a long day of work. I went not because I wanted to lose the weight but to get closer to being the kind of person I wanted to be: A healthy and strong human being who made lifestyle changes in order to respect themselves and live a life of longevity they deserved. This was the 2.0 version of me I was building, one habit at a time. I didn't always perform to my fullest, but I knew that by strength training I would be breaking down my muscles to strengthen them in the long run. Before I knew it, I would flex my arms and actually feel strong! That in itself felt good!

Ahh... food. My favorite part. This was the part I avoided for the longest. Why? Because I love food. Food was my go-to, my escape, my pleasure, and my pain. I knew when I was starting out, tackling food would be too difficult of a feat, so I left it on the sidelines for when I was ready to pick it up again. I would love to say that I feel fulfilled by eating a stick of celery slathered in a teaspoon of peanut butter, I'd love to say that basic baked chicken breast with steamed broccoli is my favorite dish to dine on, but I can't say it because this chapter is based on being authentic and true to myself. The most harm I ever did was lying to myself in any situation. Food is something I will always love, but I now choose to love it consciously. I am working on using smaller plates so I can eat smaller portions, turning off distractions such as my cell phone, Netflix, or any other noise that will distract me from my food, chewing my food slowly so I can savor every bite, and pausing to taste the aromas and flavors. Slowing down when I eat and focusing on my food makes me want to eat less. When I eat, I give my full attention to what is on my plate and not the distractions that surround me. In doing so, I hope to lessen my hunger one day at a time and through one meal at a time. There will be times where I fail, and I will smile in those moments because I now know that I can simply start again. It feels good to know that now!

So, this was a piece of me for you to savor. I'm not sure if this was what you expected or if you already knew this, and this simply served as a reminder. I just remember when I started out that there was a wealth of information out there but never enough to keep me on the path I embarked on. I often got sidetracked, and the worst part wasn't the weight gain, the lack of energy, or even endless days. It was that I couldn't stop ruminating on *why* I wasn't enough. The feeling of not being enough made me crave doing, eating, and thinking even more.

What's important is to decide if you are you choosing your life, or is your life choosing you? When you take the time to slow down, observe, and reassess, you'll be surprised to see what you have already created. Life does not stop for us, and there is no "aha" moment. Sometimes you have to take the time to realize that you need to stop and start somewhere. The gift in each moment is when you will realize that there is never a perfect moment. So you choose… now or later? Either way, it's up to you to decide. You are ENOUGH. Once you understand that, you'll never have to get over anything again. That's when you'll realize, you've had enough. The only time to begin is now because later will never come, as long as you're in the NOW.

THANK YOU

I would like to take the time to express my deepest gratitude towards my dad, stepmother, and brother. They provide me with the solid foundation to who I am today. My deepest appreciation for my great friend, Toni Rebic, as she has taught me the ability to love myself first in all life situations. My best friends, Jennifer Rozon and Shiellah Quintos, who have helped me realize new things about myself and have always been loving as well as supportive towards my dreams. My team at Starbucks, who have always had my back from day one. My wonderful landlord, Lillian, who was there for me, as I went through tough times. Even my boyfriend at the time and his family and friends, for imparting many life lessons - I would not be who I am without any of them. To all the loving friends I have not mentioned, I love you all. Thank you Ky-Lee, for giving me this opportunity to share my story with the world. It is the greatest gift you could ever give me.

~ Jy Nanda

HEALTHY SELF – "HEAL – THY" SELF

YOUR LIFE, TIME, ENERGY, THOUGHTS, AND BODY ARE PRECIOUS. PLEASE FOCUS ON YOURSELF.

by Charleyne Oulton

Charleyne Oulton

Charleyne Oulton has a passion for plant-based nutrition and a desire to make healthy eating an easy, fast, tasty, and fun habit for herself and her young family. She is a confident and happy stay at home mom of three who lives on beautiful Vancouver Island, BC. She is genuine, experienced, and passionate, and refuses to forget about her own physical and mental well-being, despite the busy and beautiful chaos of raising a family. Charleyne truly believes that being healthy is quite simple and very rewarding. She believes that when one makes quality decisions and does not quit, then they too can, and will, succeed. She is a well-established independent distributor for a health and wellness company called It Works. Charleyne is a warrior who has battled and survived depression, anxiety, an eating disorder, physical and sexual trauma, obesity, divorce, and the births of premature children who spent months in the neonatal intensive care unit (NICU). It is her purpose to inspire women, specifically the busy, overworked, and exhausted mothers around the world to find happiness, health, and harmony in their lives. Her motto: *Love yourself enough to live a healthy life.*

WWW.COACHCHARLEYBROWN.COM
ig: coach.charley.brown | fb: coachcharleybrown

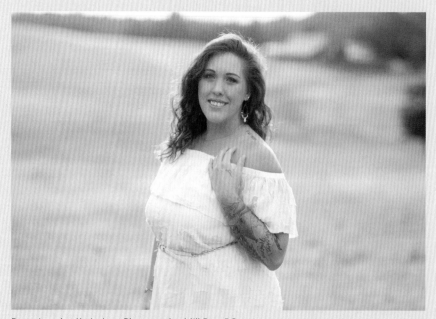

Portraiture by: Katie Jean Photography, Mill Bay, BC

The beautiful thing about life is that you can always change, grow, and manifest a positive alteration. You are not defined by your past or your prior choices. *Today* is a blessing, a new day, and a fresh start. *Today* you can start over, and today you can focus on *your* physical and mental health. I have three kids aged ten, eleven, and thirteen. As I write this, I cannot even fathom how incredibly fast time has gone by. It is so, so hard to juggle their sports schedules, school commitments, housework, my divorce, a thriving new relationship, and my online coaching job, while also focusing on my *own* health and fitness goals.

Unfortunately, if you are a mother, you probably could agree that health and self-care are usually forgotten as you find yourself taking care of everyone else around you. I was only eighteen when I had my first child. Shortly after, I delivered "Irish Twins" (well, they are thirteen months apart). [1] All my children were born premature with complex health issues. Between nursing, pumping, diaper changes, illnesses, and developmental delays, I utterly and completely let myself go. I totally got lost in the chaos of raising three kids under three. My only priority and focus was their well-being. I gave them my all. I left nothing for myself nor my spouse at the time. This is a hard lesson for any new mother. Before long, I found myself grossly overweight, extremely stressed, very unhealthy, and suffering postpartum depression, amongst GI issues. Why? Because I neglected myself.

WE MUST NOT FORGET OUR OWN SELF.

I See That Now, But I Didn't Then

The stress of my environment, along with my poor daily habits, was taking a toll on my body, spirit and mind. According to WebMD, stress is a part of life. What matters most is how you handle it. [2] With time, my kids grew. We entered the toddler years, and one day I saw myself in a photo and cried. I cried and cried; it was the first time I truly saw how much my appearance had changed. When I meditated about this later on, I came to the realization that I was most likely also suffering from postpartum depression and post-traumatic stress disorder (PTSD). I sought help, but I couldn't seem to find the right person to connect with. Doctors, counselors, psychologists, therapists, mommy groups, and online support groups - these all helped a little bit but were not addressing the root of my problem. The biggest issue in my chaos, was the fact that I was not focusing on my daily diet, staying hydrated, or getting enough sleep. I was struggling to focus on managing my stress load and neglecting my health and daily consumption.

Coach Charley Brown

At the time, I was introduced to a plant-based protein shake by some good friends. This introduction changed my life. Why? Because I started to pay attention to what I consumed, and let me tell you, I was disgusted. For the first time in my adult life, I was starting to focus on *myself*, my health, and becoming aware of what I put into my body (even though scheduling this time just for myself felt quite selfish). Within six months, I saw MASSIVE improvement. Proper nutrition, along with a very in-depth and honest relationship with both my counselor and family general practitioner (GP), is what made the biggest impact on my health. I started to keep an honest food journal and instantly knew what I could do to help myself. I started to blog and journal on social media channels by sharing my own raw experiences and routine. This was not easy, but it truly helped hold me accountable. When you bare your all on social media, you instantly try harder to do better. I participated in (and led) challenge groups. I met some like-minded and inspirational women (and men). I started to photograph and post every time I ate food (even if I was making poor choices) and also documented my own transformation. I was being real and truthful, and my friends, family, and followers loved this. I tried a few other "diets" and workouts, and soon I discovered what worked best for my body. I discovered how good being "healthy" can feel and what a positive impact it had on my life.

> "It is health that is real wealth, and not pieces of gold and silver."
> ~MAHATMA GANDHI

Today, I am happy and healthy. I'm no longer suffering from depression or struggling with stress or anxiety. I have successfully gained control of my weight and found my confidence. I am proud of my body and am in love with it, even with my curves, stretch marks, and scars. The very best part of this whole journey is that I am able to pour myself into many other women, worldwide, who are struggling to also find the time to focus on themselves. I lead by example, teaching them how to believe and fully accept themselves by reinforcing the positive. I help them cope and release their stresses and burdens and teach them how to nourish their minds, bodies, and spirits. Every single day, women and men approach me for advice, recipes, support, guidance, or inspiration. I feel so honored when they share their own personal successes and struggles with me. Together, we can push and encourage each other. I have found my tribe, and I love them fiercely. For this, I am eternally thankful.

Your life, time, energy, thoughts, and body are precious.
Please, carve out some time today just to FOCUS on YOURSELF.

As I write this, I can't help but wonder, *What have YOU done for YOURSELF today?* I beg you to carve out just a few moments just for *yourself* today! Please! *Right now.* If you need a supportive friend, I can help you get back on track both mentally and physically. But remember, I can only show you the door. You have to be the one to bravely take that first step and walk through it. I invite you to follow me on my social media, where you will find recipes and inspiration. The meals I create for my family are easy, fast, healthy, and affordable. Please listen to me when I say this, you will never regret the time and energy you pour into yourself. Yes, your kids need your attention, maybe your spouse does too. There is always work to do, and the house work is constant. But you must love yourself *and* make your physical, emotional, and mental well-being a priority through all of this gorgeous chaos.

> "You need to learn how to select your thoughts just the same way you select your clothes every day. This is a power you can cultivate. If you want to control things in your life so bad, work on the mind. That's the only thing you should be trying to control."
>
> ~ ELIZABETH GILBERT, EAT, PRAY, LOVE

Unfortunately, you don't just magically wake up in bed one morning and decide that today is the day you will fully accept and deeply love yourself, snap your fingers, have abs, and no longer crave sugar. At least, that's not how it went for me. For myself, it's still a constant internal battle against my flaws, my past, my stress patterns, my insecurities, and my determination to be healthy. I start each day by carving out a few moments in the morning to plan my day (including my meals), to drink water, and to take deep, calming breaths, because you and I both know that the day will be busy, especially if you're raising little humans like I am.

I love to cook and bake, especially with my children. I always encourage them to help me in the kitchen. They are all old enough to help me meal prep, grocery shop, wash the produce, cook or bake, and serve the meal. The whole time, we talk about the ingredients we are using, the nutrition each ingredient holds, and the kids feel so proud and excited every time they make a meal. They do not even realize the different lessons they are learning, and at the same time, they are holding me accountable. Plus, to be very honest, I truly cherish and love these precious moments with them.

One of the easiest ways for me to ensure my family and I are eating enough fruit and vegetables is to allow us to eat "picnic style." It seems so easy, and not very exciting or practical, but mark my words, we will all see a huge increase in our daily produce if it's washed, chopped up, and ready to be eaten in single serving portions. This is so easy to take and eat as we drive to lacrosse, gymnastics, or hockey. We have something healthy to snack on while we do homework, feel an urge to snack, or are cuddled up watching a movie. If I don't meal prep when the kids are in school, then we are more likely to fail at healthy eating that evening. So, typically,

I will prep dinner and an after school picnic as soon as I get home from school drop off. You do not need to spend thousands of dollars every month to fully nourish yourself and your family. I am a huge fan of using what you already have in your fridge, freezer, pantry, and garden. Sometimes the kids' after school picnic includes raisins or other dried fruits, something freshly baked, or something on a kabob. I basically work with what I have available at home.

For those of you who may not always have a fridge, freezer, or a pantry full of healthy and nourishing ingredients, I encourage you to learn what resources and programs are available in your community. Locally, we have community gardens for those who do not have a home garden. We have the "good food box program" that you can sign up for. Additionally, you could always start your own or join a neighborhood, school, or community "produce swap." I also love to shop at local markets in the spring and summer; I find this a very afford-able way to load up on produce and help sup-port our neighbors. I try to add fresh fruit to each and every meal, for each and every one of us. Sometimes it's quinoa salad with blueber-ries on the side or a clean protein source with baked yams and fresh sliced watermelon. Other times, it's seeds or nuts with broccoli and a leafy salad. I know it sounds silly and strange to have fruit with dinner, but somehow, it always tastes great. Plus, it really helps with my budget

You do not need to spend thousands of dollars every month to fully nourish yourself and your family. I am a huge fan of using what you already have in your fridge, freezer, pantry, and garden.

as we use what is already on hand, while adding extra enzymes, vitamins, and min-erals to our meal. I only discovered quinoa about four years ago, and now it is a sta-ple in my house. We love quinoa and eat it with many of our meals. Quinoa is gluten-free, high in protein, and one of the few plant foods that contain all nine es-sential amino acids. [3] I add cooked and cooled quinoa to most of our dinners. Some-times I mix it with a cup of rice or add a cup to pasta sauces or salads. A few spoonfuls of cooked and cooled quinoa tastes great mixed with yogurt in the morn-ings, and sometimes I'll sneak it into our shakes and smoothies, too. My favorite way to serve it is mixed with fresh, homemade greek salad. Mmmm. Believe it or not, after time the human body naturally craves good, clean nutrition.

Let's Talk About Morning Routines

My kids used to wake up and wander all sleepy-eyed and adorable into my bedroom almost every day. Typically, they would fall back asleep in my bed or lay there talking to each other and petting the dog or kittens whilst slowly waking up. Now, I'm raising preteens, and it takes time to get them out of bed and showered. Then, we all get ready and head downstairs. Together, we make healthy lunches (for mom too!), check the calendar, talk about after-school sports, and pack their backpacks (and re-pack them…). All of this takes *time*. One time-saving meal solution in our house is to make a smoothie or protein shake for us all to share and enjoy. I love shakes and smoothies because they can be all natural and are loaded with vitamins, proteins, vegetables and fruit; they're healthy, delicious, and fast! I love to add a scoop of our supplement shake mix and tons of fresh or frozen fruit (and don't forget veggies too). When I buy fresh local fruit or fruit on sale, I often divide it in half: half to freeze and half to enjoy now. To freeze, I lay the washed and dried produce on a cookie sheet lined with parchment, spread it out, and freeze. Once frozen, I add this to our shakes! Avocado, berries, melons, banana, kale, and spinach: these all freeze wonderfully, and, once added to a smoothie, really make it cold and creamy. Do not forget about herbs and spices; we often add vanilla, cinnamon, nutmeg, cloves, basil, or cilantro to our smoothies for that extra flavor and nutrition.

It took me eighteen months to lose the 95 pounds I gained while pregnant. I've managed to keep it off for over three years now. I tried the shakes and loved them. I tried the women only gym, I paid for a personal trainer (that I did not use). I bought the at-home workout DVDs too. I found pros and cons with all of this. I've run countless kilometers both on a treadmill and outside.

I love to explore, geocache, and hike through trails on our amazing island. I crave time outside, unplugged, alone and in nature. I walk. I've dabbled in hot yoga, swam laps, and also tried (and loved) Crossfit. I've learned that *I like it all* and cannot seem to commit to just one of the above. I like and crave change, and this works for me, especially with my chaotic mom schedule. I used to find every excuse in the world to *not* reach my goals: "I'm too busy," "I'm too tired," and "The house needs to be cleaned." If you can relate to these words, these thoughts, or this pattern, I beg you to stop what you're doing right now and say out loud: "Today, I will love myself, and I will eat healthy and exercise!" Stop focusing on your weaknesses or insecurities; it's not going to get you anywhere in life. If you want to change, if you want to be successful, if you want to get healthier, and if you want to lose fat and gain muscle, then it's time to start seeing and focusing on your unique strengths and celebrate them! Focus on what you are good at, what you enjoy, and find a way to incorporate this into your weekly routine.

> "Take care of your body. It's the only place you have to live."
> ~ JIM ROHN

Decide on some short and long term goals. Make a list. Write them out, seriously. Short term goals can be as simple as this:

- DRINK ONE glass of water every hour I am awake today
- NO pop or alcohol today
- Quit smoking
- SMILE today
- Choose to be positive with my words and actions
- EAT BREAKFAST (fresh fruit, a smoothie or shake, oatmeal)
- WALK more today
- EAT the rainbow, not the sugary candy, but a variety of produce
- SLEEP eight hours tonight

I repeat this affirmation daily, and encourage you to try it as well: "I am going to control what I can and I am not going to lose peace of mind over what I can not." YOU are amazing, unique, beautiful, and worthy of your time, love, and attention. Once you start to believe this, you will discover a new confidence and appreciation of yourself and gain an inner knowing and deep understanding that you are capable of greatness and of accomplishing your goals, including eating healthier and establishing a new routine. You've got this! Nourish your body with positive thoughts and healthy nutrients. Not only do you deserve the very best in life, your body does as well.

Remember, it's just going to take a change in the way you behave, think, and view yourself, a fresh start. The moment to start taking action is right now. I believe in you. Now it's your turn to believe in yourself. If I can find happiness, health, confidence, and joy while juggling three children, a divorce, health issues, a booming online coaching company, and a new relationship then why the hell can't you? What's your excuse? Time to cut the bullshit. Realize your worth. Be kind to yourself.

Much Love,
Charleyne Oulton
#coachcharleybrown

THANK YOU

Jeff, Libby, Kathy, Jerry, Jason, Lisa, Les, Shelley, Madeleine, Jonathan, Jenn, Heather, Courtney, Cindy, Chaentelle, Bea, Sandy, Mike, Trish, Kim, Katie, Samantha, Kristen. I found my courage and confidence because of your constant encouragement.
~ Charleyne Oulton

MINDFUL LIVING FOR THE EMPOWERED WOMAN

"AT ANY GIVEN TIME, WE ARE BEING MINDFUL OR MINDLESS. THERE IS NO OTHER WAY."

by Kelly Spencer

(ret.) Registered Nurse, RN
Certified Yoga Teacher, CYT
Certified Life Coach

Kelly Spencer

Kelly Spencer is a mindful life enthusiast, living each day as it comes. Retiring early as a registered nurse, Kelly made the shift into holistic wellness over twenty years ago. As an entrepreneur, certified life coach, yoga and meditation teacher, and writer, Kelly demonstrates the capacity to live your life in awareness and at the same time in tune with your own inner mission and vision. She truly lives by the quote from Gandhi: "Be the change you wish to see in the world."

Kelly shares with others her ability to think critically while having an open heart and mind with a side of humor. She doesn't take life too seriously and enjoys an herbal tea as much as a beer. She is the perfect display of balance and creativity. Extremely daring and ready to take on life with all its twists and turns, Kelly's open minded, loving, and passionate nature can be seen in everything she does and in her interactions with the people she encounters. Her honest and compassionate outlook and deep connection to nature, the elements, and all living things have assisted her own personal journey of healing and growth. She now follows her calling as an author where she shares her unique insights about universal truths with a much wider audience through her weekly column, her periodic publications in highly acclaimed magazines, such as *The Elephant Journal* or through co-authoring and authoring books. She is a charismatic and creative spirit with real life experiences that give meaning to her words. She inspires all that cross her path to take responsibility for their lives through self-leadership.

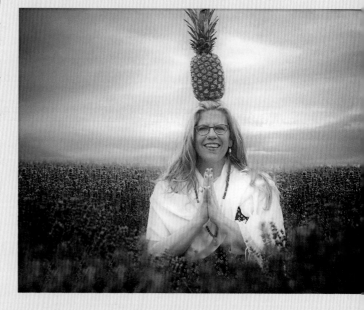

Kelly believes in the magic that exists in the world and in each one of us.

WWW.KELLYMSPENCER.COM
ig: indigolounge
fb: manduukii.kellyspencer

Your workout is complete, and your to-do list is done. You throw your feet up to watch your favorite Netflix binge of the moment, and hungry-boredom sets in. As a "treat," you decide to grab a handful of chips from the bag that you've stashed in the top corner of the cupboard. Before you get to episode number three of back-to-back viewing, the entire bag of chips is void, leaving only a salty, guilty crumb-blanket on your lap. Licking your fingers one by one, you consider the empty bag, pondering where you can get more, while also wondering how the heck that just happened.

> "Many people are alive but don't touch the miracle of being alive."
>
> ~ THICH NHAT HANH

Fifteen years ago, I was hospitalized and unable to breathe. My heart rate was dangerously low and irregular, and my body was fevered and achy. I had a very fragile gut on any given day with heart burn, acidity and irregularity, but with this mystery illness I had contracted, I was violently ill. It was really no surprise to be so physically devastated and inflicted, as my body, mind, and spirit had bottomed out some time ago.

In more mild states, I was sick often and found myself frequently making doctors' appointments. I ate processed food that was destroying my gastrointestinal enzymes. The abundance of meat, wheat, and dairy I consumed had me in an acidic agony and wreaked hormonal havoc. I worked a job that was extremely stressful and carried that stress around with me like it was some sort of prized luxury name brand bag. I was going through a fevered divorce from a diseased marriage. My children, contaminated by the dysfunction that had become our routine norm, were equally ailing. Seemingly so, my body was just catching up to pace and the crisis that made me end up in the hospital for a week hooked up to electrodes, heart monitors, intravenous therapy, and oxygen prongs was my wake-up call. I had been constantly living in the past, replaying and replaying the dysfunctions of my life. The ones I didn't preview obsessively, I ignored, denied, or minimized. I anesthetized my personal stress and discomforts with unhealthy choices.

As a registered nurse, I was used to taking care of others. That moment when they put the ECG heart monitor on me at the hospital, and I saw the erratic blip of my existence with a heart rate of only thirty-eight beats per minute, I knew it was time to become more mindful, start a new chapter, and take care of myself.

Mindfulness is a state of active awareness and attention on the present moment. When we are being mindful, we observe the thoughts and feelings we are experiencing right now. Using our minds by witnessing and observing with detachment allows us to let go of judging our thoughts and feelings, as good or bad. It is important to let go of judgments, as this can welcome unwanted emotions such as guilt or shame.

In an age where we are connected to everything (and frequently) through our phones, internet, and social media, we are constantly interrupted and pulled externally. When we practice mindful living, we create an inward action of returning to our centre. It is about having eyes wide open to what is genuinely going on within us and surrounding us. This consciousness (or lack of) affects the choices we make in our health and with our environment. We are the most empowered source of knowledge and expertise about the decisions we make as individual holistic beings, regarding our own health.

Being mindful is the single most powerful thing we can do for our well-being. As women, we can access the benefits of mindful living to enhance the health of our mind-body connection and to bring appreciation of our culinary choices and the benefits of conscious food consumption. Although we are multi-tasking machines, it's crucial for us to live intently and with focus. Tapping into the mindful attention of the present moment allows us to actively participate in decisions that decrease our stress levels and promote health and happiness. Leading a mindfulness lifestyle is a powerful tool for us as individuals, as well the environment and collective consciousness.

Stress

Bruce H. Lipton, PhD, an internationally recognized leader and stem cell biologist reports findings that show 95% of all illness or dis-ease (the lack of ease) are the result of stress. According to American Institute of Stress, the consequences of stress-related illnesses, from depression to heart disease, costs businesses an estimated $200 to $300 billion a year in lost productivity. In a male dominated business world, the number one killer in men, is stress in the form of cardiovascular incidents, heart attack, and stroke. [1] Historically, women were much lower on this statistical list. That is until gender equality was fairly implemented. Unfortunately for women, as we begin to implement more equal opportunity for jobs, it means equal opportunity for stress related diseases.

When we are stressed, a hormone called cortisol can become elevated. It is often referred to as the "stress hormone." This elevation creates a whole series of undesirable effects on our body and mind. Elevated cortisol levels can increase gastric acid production, which if chronic, can lead to reflux and other problems in the intestine, creating digestive difficulties. This agitates the reproductive system, creating challenges such as disruption of normal ovulation and menstrual cycles, difficulty getting pregnant or carrying a pregnancy, and also infertility. When our reproductive system declines in function, unfortunately our testosterone levels can also deplete. This can play havoc not only with our Goddess parts, but with our muscle mass and fitness goals.

Stress also seems to affect food choices we are making. We know through multiple studies (and experience) that physical or emotional distress can increase our appetite for intake of foods high in fat and / or sugar. Not only can stress and lack of mindfulness steer us down the wrong grocery aisle, but it can be the culprit of overeating, and therefore weight gain. For some, stress creates a loss of appetite and can leave us depleted of vital nutrition and hydration that is essential for our integrated wellness. When we are stressed we also tend to lose sleep, exercise less, and drink more alcohol, all of which can contribute to keeping us from our healthiest and happiest versions of ourselves.

Be Aware, Let It Go. Reach Higher

Did you know that our emotional response to each moment directly affects our DNA? Did you know that the body houses trillions of DNA cells? Studies have found that the power of intentional thought and emotion directly affect our cells.[2] Each time we allow ourselves to mindlessly stay in low vibrational states (such as anger, fear, and stress overload), trillions of DNA cells have objectionable effects. Fortunately, once we shift to intentional high vibrational states of thought and feeling (such as gratitude, love, and compassion) the DNA responds favorably. Our emotions and our DNA responses may be creating favorable responses in our bodies which might be the difference between hair growth versus hair loss, deep sleep or insomnia, happy gut or irritable bowel syndrome.

Energy In Must Equate To Energy Out

Some of the biggest energy vacuums are negative emotions and stress. On a cellular level, our bodies store our experiences within our physical frame and it's imperative we release what does not serve us. By taking care of our stress levels through mindfulness activities that connect us to our whole multifaceted self, such as yoga, meditation, or a brisk, observant walk in the woods, we empower ourselves and equate the energies in our life. We make smarter food choices and create an optimal internal gastrointestinal system. We also support happy hormones, create favorable cellular responses, and a content state of holistic wellness. Be aware of your stress levels - release your stress in a way that serves you well and then reach higher to a thought, feeling or action that expands you.

Some of the biggest energy vacuums are negative emotions and stress.

A diet that is local, organic, non-GMO (non-genetically modified) and primarily plant-based (foods that can be grown such as beans, legumes, fruits, vegetables, seeds, nuts and herbs) creates an homeostatic state that the body seeks to maintain. This ideal, mindful, and conscious way to fuel with food creates a condition of balance within and even reduces and / or eliminates disease.

Eating whole foods with minimal processing or refinement, which are free from additives or other artificial substances such as artificial sweeteners, MSG, high-fructose corn syrup, and food dyes are utilized more efficiently by our bodies. By providing the smart nutrients for our internal systems, we function more effectively and support the mind in achieving clarity and focus.

We have all heard the importance of drinking plenty of water each day. Dr. Masura Emoto, a Japanese scientist has taken this importance to an all new dimension with his water research findings. [3] Dr. Emoto has proven that how we feel and the energy we emit can directly affect water cells. His published work shows the drastic and profound difference of a water cell exposed to "hate" versus one surrounded in the energy of "love." Our body's constitution is 70% water, so one can conclude that the cells within our body also have a diverse reaction to the polarity of feelings we experience. Tell your water how much you love and appreciate it, it will literally change you both.

The same gratitude and lovefest can be directed to your food. Before you consume anything, keep in mind that food can contain a high level of H2O as well. Some of my favorite foods are zucchini, celery, and radish—they are 90% water! So, the next time you drink a glass of water and have a bite to eat, think of something or someone you love and are grateful for: The power of positivity changes the water molecules ingested and the cells within you!

Just Breathe

One of the easiest and quickest ways to connect the body and mind, is to stop, close your eyes, and take 3-10 minutes of slow, rhythmic breaths in through the nose and out through the nose. If you are really feeling the need to release, let the exhale be an audible pronounced exhale through the mouth. Mindful breath work creates an instant body-mind connection. The focus of breathing allows the mind to focus on the present moment, your breath, and slowly quiet down from the hundreds of thoughts swirling and the constant pull to external forces. Mindful breathing facilitates a few moments of spending quality time with yourself—your body, your mind, your thoughts and feelings—and it provides an opportunity to really honor the present moment.

Your mind will wander, and stress will creep back in. The goal is not to completely quiet the mind, but try and focus on the breath. Deeper breaths, a calmer and more mindful thought process will create a higher oxygen delivery to our cells and a beneficial response on the cells.

Use quiet time in the ladies' room or set a small soothing timer on your phone each hour to remind yourself to check in, take inventory of the current state of your body and mind and take some slow, deep breaths. It is with this inventory awareness of what is, as is, that we can assume authentic action in the direction of what is best for our own health.

Mindful movement is any physical movement that we bring intentional awareness too. Hiking a mountain can be mindful. Going for a run can be too. Mindfulness practices are not just solely reserved for yoga, Tai Chi, and meditation. Any practice that requires deliberate and designed objectives for the body and mind to work together and brings forth an awareness of the powerful connection within that relationship is a mindfulness practice.

Collective Consciousness & The Environment

Whether we eat vegetarian, omnivore, or plant-based, the choices we make have a direct impact on the world, our fellow humans, and the natural elements of the earth. Our chosen diet should be local as much as possible, fair-trade, organic or no chemical spray, non-GMO (non-genetically modified), and primarily plant-based. Whether you eat meat or not, vegetables should be the main attraction on your plate and 80% of your food should be plant-based foods that are grown sustainably. As stated, this creates a homeostatic state not only for the body, but also for the rest of the world.

The difference in greenhouse gas emissions for animal-based versus plant-based foods is well known. 4 The amount of meat consumed, especially land-intensive agricultural products like beef, has an alarming amount of detrimental effect of our environment. A plethora of research shows us not only is (over) consumption of meat not healthy for our bodies, it is harming to our planet. Factory farming has taken over to meet the demands of meat consumption. In a hope to create revenue at a pace that keeps up to the consumer, the evolution of this farming is the eradication of the well-being of all of us, including our planet. If you choose to eat meat, eat it sparingly. Make sure it is organic, hormone-free, and antibiotic-free. Ensure it is kept with the laws of nature in mind, meaning animals are fed their native diets, not a mix of genetically modified grains and animal by-products. Look for compassionate farm practices adopting methods that recognize animal sentience (awareness of thoughts and feelings) and that give full regard to the animals' needs to live cage-free and have free-range access to the outdoors for fresh air, sunlight, and freedom.

The Food You Eat Has An Environmental Impact

The healthiest known communities on earth have a mindful diet preference that is plant-based with occasional fish. But even fish can be fishy. Aquaculture or factory farmed fish are full of chemical and dyes. [5] Through this processing, the transfer of sea lice from fish farms to juvenile wild salmon during out-migration occurs. To control this, farmers use more chemicals. For example, SLICE®, is a chemical added to salmon feed. As it is digested, it passes into the salmon's tissues and is then absorbed by any attached lice which die shortly after.

Alternatively, fish caught by trawling, which involves dragging fishnets along the ocean floor, can have three times the greenhouse gas emissions of fish caught by traditional methods. [6] So, how can we swim upstream into this dilemma? If you eat fish, go fishing. If this doesn't float your boat, then purchase fresh wild-caught fish or look for canned salmon labeled "Alaskan" or "Sockeye", as it is not permitted to be farmed.

Pay Attention To How Your Food Was Grown
And The Conditions For Those Growing It

Being mindful of the impact our food has on our water, earth, and air is imperative. Genetically modified organisms (GMO) in our crops and food affect our health as well as our entire ecosystem. Bees are crucial in the pollination of many food crops, but are unfortunately extremely endangered due to modern agricultural techniques, such as GMO crops. [7]

When we are choosing food consciously and ethically, we should also consider the people that are farming it. Fair Trade is a transparency and respect based trading agreement that seeks greater equity in international trade. It ensures farmers get a fair price for their crops—the most common being cocoa, coffee, bananas, tea, and sugar — and must be free of forced labor or poor working conditions for laborers. The crops are raised through sustainable methods, and no genetically modified crops can be certified fair trade.

We Are The Sacred Nurturers Of Life And Our Planet

When the timing is right or when we require togetherness, my bestie and I have date night; we leave all other obligations at home and we romance and nurture the important collective women consciousness. There is a good meal prepared, a nice wine poured, and an exchange of the frustrations and celebrations we are experiencing in our lives. There are always lots of laughs and occasionally some tears.

When looking back in history, we see strong sisterhood, women circles, and a close relationship between women spending time together. Time for exchanging experiences and wisdom, opportunity for embracing our feminine energy and building the importance of time spent with each other.

We are our biggest cheerleaders and champion of the rights of all. We are sisters of an empowered clan of sisterhood with an etheric cord of connection strung together. We feel our plights and struggles, as well as our loves and joys, with deep compassion. When we let go of our own self-judgment, subsequent judgment and competition with each other, we are truly Goddesses: intelligent, funny, compassionate, giving, appreciative, and beautiful. When we empower ourselves, we give each other permission to do the same. By living mindfully, we create a healthy and happy platform for ourselves and as the sacred nurturers of life and our planet.

Act on it. Step into the change you want through authentic action.

Write down in your journal these headings:
- Mindful Eating and Conscious Consumption
- Mindful Body-Mind Connection & Movement
- Mindful Stress Levels & Energy Management
- Mindful Environment: People & The Earth

Under each title list three ways you can live more mindfully in this area of your life. Beside each new mindful action, write one or two ways you will create and obtain this. Update your list each New Moon (every twenty-eight days) with gratitude and celebration for every small step you have taken.

For example, under, "Mindful Eating and Conscious Consumption," you might write: I will start to buy more organic and local food by:
- Investigating local farmers markets
- Reading food labels to ensure organic and non-GMO

Happiness Is An Inside Job

Over the last decade and a half, I have learned and studied how becoming more knowledgeable and mindful in all areas of our life, can assist us to be happier and healthy. I picked one of these areas to focus on at a time and when I felt ready, I added a new source of mindfulness. Life still has stressors, however, I watch what I eat by eating foods that suit me best, I meditate regularly, and I am happy to say that I haven't been to a doctor for over a decade. Ultimately, how mindfully or mindlessly we are participating in this experience of life is up to us.

THANK YOU

A mindful shout out to my children. Since the day they were born, I have viewed the world through their eyes. They have influenced me to be more present and to nurture mindfulness. They have inspired me to be healthier - body, mind, and spirit. My desire for them to live their best life continually motivates me to live the best version of my life.

~ Kelly Spencer

FIT ON HER PLATE

Featuring

Ashly Hill

Deirdre Slattery

Paula Man

Neli Hession

HIGH INTENSITY FOR THE INTENSE WOMAN

LIMITATIONS ARE FEAR
IN ITS MOST CONTROLLING FORM.
YOUR WILL TO CHANGE IS THE STRENGTH
TO BREAK THROUGH THEM!

by Ashly Hill

Bachelor of Science, BSc
Minor in Kinesiology (MKin)
Minor in Psychology (MPsy)
Personal Trainer, PT

Ashly Hill

Ashly is a kinesiologist who holds a degree in both kinesiology and psychology and has devoted her life to helping others achieve total wellness. Her career in the health and fitness industry started when she became a receptionist for an independent gym in New Westminster. She was very eager to learn and advanced quickly by becoming a certified personal trainer within six months. However, due to being so successful at such a young age, she struggled to earn the respect of her colleagues. This was not going to hold her back though. Her passion for anatomy and physiology grew even more while she studied Sports Science at Douglas College. After two years at Douglas College, she received admission into Simon Fraser University, where she immersed herself in as many health and fitness industries as possible.

She worked as a conditioning coach for division 1 & 2 youth soccer players, as a personal trainer in the corporate gym world. She began to establish herself as an independent trainer by holding boot camps in local parks and training clients at local community centers, and even finished her final year at SFU while working as an as-sistant office manager in a multidisci-plinary clinic. However, she really found her niche working in management. Post graduation, she worked as the general operating manager for a local Vancouver, B.C fitness studio, Fit In 30 Minutes. It was then, that she was able to be proud of her accomplishments by passing her experi-ence and knowledge on to her team so they could be the best coaches possible.

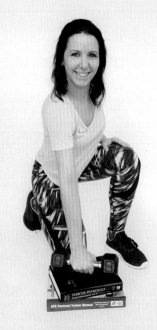

ig: ashly_health | li: ashly-hill

Swapping Life Intensity For School Intensity For High Intensity

In order for you to fully understand where my passion towards a healthy life stems from, I am going to have to share some personal stories from my past. This is not easy, so bear with me. At a very young age, I grew up in a household where stability was not that common. I moved around a lot, so much so, that I attended over fifteen schools and never made it past the ninth grade. Most of the adults in my life smoked heavily and drank alcohol on a regular basis. I was barely in grade eight when I started to use marijuana. They say marijuana is a gateway drug, and in my case, they were right. The instability that I was used to began to cascade into my own personal decisions. I was skipping school, using recreational drugs, and blatantly did not have a care in the world for responsibilities. My father was not in the picture and although my mother tried her best to contain my rebellious behavior, I was in a whirlwind of disobedience, rebellion, and self destruction. I was expelled from school, which only pushed me further into the life of drug use and partying. In an attempt to move me away from all that, my mother and I moved from British Columbia, Canada to Ontario, Canada. Her attempt was not successful, in fact, I only got worse. After struggling with addiction and insecurities from my childhood up until I was in my early twenties, one day I had an awakening. Was I going to go down the path that made me just another statistic for Census Canada, end up in jail or more likely, dead? I knew I was stronger than that, I knew it was time to break tradition.

I remember it very clearly as if it was yesterday. I was in my best friend's car driving to some unrecalled destination when I made the decision to go back to school. I didn't have anyone advising me to go, or better yet, I didn't even know if it was the right decision, but I did know that I felt like it was the only way I could escape from the bubble I was trapped in. I turned to my friend and asked her, "I really want to go to school for something because I think it's going to help me get out of this chaotic life I'm living, but I have no idea what to take. Any ideas?" She turned to me and said with such confidence, "You need to take something in anatomy, Ashly. You love sports and the human body so much; it's your industry, it's where you are meant to be!" It was from that time forward that I started making moves and I have not looked back since. Learning about the body, how the mind grows and develops from our environment, and the barriers that hold us back from becoming the best that we can truly be, was my anti-drug. It gives me immense pleasure to be able to impact other people's lives and if there is anyway that I can make a change, I will.

I was a full-time student for seven years and during that time, I juggled a part-time job, and the daily responsibilities of adulthood. Since I was independent and lived on my own, I tried to have a social life. What I did not make time for was any form of physical activity. How could I, someone who was an advocate for health and wellness, even consider using the same excuse that I scolded so many others for making? Clearly, I was not practicing what I preached, even knowing full well that the common excuse, "I don't have enough time" was unacceptable. After sitting for countless hours day in and day out, tirelessly studying to retain literature, I started to experience the effects of inactivity: sore hips, back pain, and fatigue. The pain lingered and progressively got worse; it began to affect me in such a way that I was losing sleep. I couldn't study for more than a few hours at a time without my back spasming, and I no longer had the ability to pay attention in lectures. I decided enough was enough and that something had to be done.

It was roughly the third year into my degree when I made a change. I had always preferred fast-paced activities and knew that I would only ever be able to fit 30–40 minutes of exercise into my busy schedule. I had to be in and out in under an hour for it to fit. However, short resistance routines were just not cutting it, I wasn't losing much body fat and I sure as hell didn't want the "freshman 15." I started designing my workouts in such a way that included circuits of high intensity cardio paired with 12–15 repetitions of weight training exercises: a style of training now known as high intensity functional training (HIFT). HIFT became my only means of activity, and within six months I had completely eliminated my back pain, I regained my energy levels, and with constant stretching, my hips no longer were restricted. Once I became a personal coach, I carried my newfound style of training into the routines I designed for my clients, and they loved it! Not only did it work, but who couldn't fit a short twenty to thirty minute workout into their schedule? A simple solution to the common barrier of having "no time" has now become my passion and career.

Priorities

When you first wake up in the morning, what is the first thing you do? If you are like most people, you likely check social media, look at your calendar, and read your emails. At some point in your day, do you find yourself scrolling through Pinterest looking for that new recipe to use for dinner; skimming through photos that you've seen a hundred times? Because I do. At any point in your day, do you prioritize your health? When it comes to health and fitness, the most common excuse is, "I don't have enough time." What if I told you, all you need is thirty minutes? Would you be able to find 30 minutes out of the

Would you be able to find 30 minutes out of the 1,440 minutes you have every day, to prolong your life?

1,440 minutes you have every day, to prolong your life?

Evolution of HIFT

High intensity functional training; also known as HIFT, are short intense work-outs that have become more popular in modern day society. The health and fitness industry— more specifically the personal training industry —has made way for a faster, more efficient, effective and exhilarating style of workout. When you con-sider the traditional methods of personal training, exhausting images of exercise —rest — exercise — rest are most likely to appear. The faster paced lifestyle we are challenged with today needed a new training style that was of the same speed and efficiency. How are we supposed to fit an hour workout in between work, kids, and day-to-day responsibilities? The common response would be, *I can't.* In order to overcome the barrier of "no time," there needed to be a shift in the culture of fit-ness training, which ultimately paved the way for HIFT.

HIFT merged the traditional methods of cardiovascular and anaerobic exercise into a shorter workout. Cardio and weights all in one! An example of such an exer-cise would be a dumbbell burpee to a dumbbell press. This compound exercise con-ditions the body's cardiovascular system while also incorporating resistance from the dumbbells. Using exercises like this when designing a fitness routine meant the stubborn belly fat would disappear and there would be an increase in lean muscle mass, all within a shorter workout. What could be better than that? Studies indi-cate that HIFT training, done only three times a week, could significantly improve the ability of skeletal muscle and the whole body to oxidize fats. [1] Your body needs to oxidize stored fat in order for it to be used to create energy. This meant, HIFT worked! Most importantly, HIFT training continues to work for up to forty-eight hours after you workout. [2] Your body continues to burn off that unwanted fat for more than a day and a half after your session. Without getting into the nitty gritty science on how this happens, your body needs to recover after each workout and it is this recovery process that continues to burn energy. The entire recovery pro-cess is composed of many different systems that need to return back to their orig-inal state, removal of lactic acid (the chemical that causes that burning sensation in your muscles), replenishment of the energy producing molecule adenosine tri-phosphate (also known as ATP), and the replenishment of the body's oxygen supply. This specific effect is called the exercise post oxygen consumption (EPOC) and is why HIFT surpasses other training styles in it's effectiveness of body fat reduction.

Why HIFT Was Made For Women

You may be asking yourself: how is HIFT beneficial for women specifically? Well, let me blow your mind and introduce a small, but not so tiny, statement that will start this section off properly. Heart disease is the leading cause of death in American women. [3] This is a statistic that most women aren't even aware of! Heart disease is only one form of cardiovascular disease (CVD) and is caused by a dysfunction of the cardiovascular system, a problem with that beautiful beating heart we all are trying to protect. The CVD that I am referring to, is the restriction of oxygen and nutrients to the heart caused by blocked blood vessels. [4] In today's society we are bombarded with promotional broadcasts of quick fixes since it fits right into the busy life of someone who doesn't have time. By quick fixes, I refer to corrective surgeries or prescription medication, however, what these broadcasts so devilishly leave out is that though these fixes may be quick, they are in no way permanent. The only way to truly battle such a devastating condition and keep yourself healthy for your family and children is through lifestyle changes, such as HIFT!

Ask yourself this, in the past twenty-four hours alone, how many tasks have you accomplished? The average woman juggles a career, family, and social life all within a single day. During those twenty-four hours, did you, at any point, make time for your personal health and wellness? A by-product of women being multitasking superheroes is that we tend to push the importance of our own physical health aside while catering to everyone and everything around us, thus leading us into the downward spiral of a sedentary lifestyle. Ultimately, it is the lack of physical activity that leads to a myriad of health issues such as CVD (cardiovascular disease). HIFT training will easily reverse two leading risk factors that cause CVD: large waist/hip ratio (ratio of the circumference of the waist to that of the hips), and physical inactivity. [5] Adding an hour and a half of HIFT training into your weekly routine could save your life. Do I have your attention yet?

HIFT In All Its Glory

Still wondering what a HIFT workout looks like? On this topic alone, I could write my own novel, however, I have been tasked with explaining such an intricate style in only one chapter. So, with that being said, here I go. A traditional HIFT session includes exercises that will push you to your limit. This means, exerting 110% effort! Yes, this sounds daunting, but it only lasts a short amount of time; just enough time for you to almost convince yourself you can't do it, but not so long that it prevents your inner prowess from overpowering and pushing through. That inner feline is given time to rest because the high energy bursts are followed by much easier movements that allow you to catch your breath. Don't let this fool you though, at no point did I say complete rest! You will continue to move throughout the entire workout. The type of rest used in HIFT is called active rest, where instead of sitting to catch your breath, you continue to move. Incorporating this into a workout will aid your recovery and reduce the delayed onset of muscle soreness. [6] One minute you may be asked to do twenty burpees where the next you are doing a step-up with a shoulder press holding weights in your hands. That inner voice questions your movements and you ask yourself, *Am I pushing weights or is this cardio?* That's the best part, it's both! I could go on and on about what a HIFT session looks like, however, the unique intricacy of its design is what makes having an educated instructor so important. Let them be the creative ones and let yourself focus on getting your life back! However, if spending money on a coach is not ideal, but you still want to make a change in your activity levels, these types of sessions can be conducted not just in a personal training studio, they can also be done in your house or the neighborhood park: just about anywhere you can perform a squat. That's right, the world is your oyster, so get out there and HIFT!

You Were Made To HIFT

High intensity functional training sounds like it may only be designed for the young, athletic, or physically conditioned individual, however, I can tell you now, that is entirely misleading. HIFT can be done by EVERYONE, which is why it's considered to be so versatile. Let's focus on the outliers of the female society: pregnant, postpartum and elderly women.

Pregnant women make up approximately 10% of the members at Fit In 30, in fact, we had trainers who specialized in prenatal and postpartum training. What was traditionally recognized as common knowledge —pregnant women refraining from exercise— is not so common anymore. Pregnant women are encouraged to continue the fitness regime they were doing before pregnancy, and in fact, the Society of Obstetricians and Gynecologists of Canada (SOGC) emphasize the risks of not exercising during pregnancy at all. [7] Therefore, even if you did not have a regular fitness regime before conception there is no time like the present to begin one, especially when it betters the development of your unborn child. When a woman becomes pregnant she feels bouts of heightened motivation now that she is responsible for another life. This new perception towards life is the exact saturation of hope, determination, and passion that drives her to make lifestyle changes, such as starting an exercise routine. Changes like this should be encouraged and exercise of any sort for pregnant women, that will have no contraindication, will only be beneficial for the mother and her fetus. However a consultation with a physician should always precede the start of a new fitness program. [8] As I said before, I am not here to only

113

focus on the young, as of 2016, according to Census Canada, seniors now outweigh the number of children in our population. [9]

If this statistic speaks to you, I am here to tell you that you have not been forgotten. HIFT training was also meant for you! Females are challenged with a myriad of barriers as we get into our elderly years, some of which start in our early fifties. Barriers such as fatigue and menopause, are much too life changing to disregard. Menopause is a whirlwind of unwanted physical changes: hot flashes, mood swings, weight gain, and in some cases, osteoporosis. [10] I am definitely not telling you that HIFT is a cure to these ailments, however, I will tell you that HIFT can slow the onset of some of these ailments, and make living with others more manageable. Research has shown that the combination of high impact training and resistance training is highly effective in preserving the spine in postmenopausal women. More specifically, it is more effective than either type of training on its own. This is quite different from the previous advice of walking 30 minutes a day. Saving your bones is not the only thing that HIFT can do for you. Something that we as women are all too accepting of is our mood swings. One day we wake up as happy as a kid in a candy store and the next we have to dig deep in the shadows of our own thoughts to even pull ourselves out of bed. Is this normal? No, in fact, we don't actually enjoy feeling this way. Now add menopause on top of that and you are the she-devil from hell. HIFT can aid in leveling out these mood swings by providing beneficial effects on anxiety, depression, sleep quality, and other general mood effects experienced by menopause. [9] Don't let the words "high intensity" veer you away from trying this style of training. Worried that you may not have enough energy for a workout? I'm happy to share that HIFT requires less overall energy than traditional exercise of lower to moderate intensity and with the right coach, each session will be personalized to your current level of fitness. [11]

Making Your Way To HIFT

Now that you know what HIFT is, where it can be conducted, and that you too are made for it, the next step is to find a HIFT expert. As this style becomes more popular within the training industry, you will see more and more coaches shifting their sessions into shorter more intense workouts. My advice to you is, ask any coach that you are considering hiring, exactly what their sessions look like. Since you are the client, you are fully entitled to shop around until you find exactly what you are looking for. To help guide you in what to expect, I have provided an example introductory HIFT session for you to use as a guideline.

walkouts with toe touches	x 20
mountain climbers	x 20
squats	x 20
jumping Jacks	x 20
repeat twice	

with a 6lb ball

wide opening ups	x 15
squat with press	x 15
woodchops	x 10 each side
balancing curls on one leg	x 15
balancing press on one leg	x 15
mountain climbers on a stool	x 30 sec
repeat twice	

modified pull-ups	x 15
push-ups on bench or floor	x 10
repeat twice	

knee tucks on a bench	x 20
crunches on a bench	x 20
bench squats	x 20
repeat twice	

Now you are ready to find your very own HIFT coach or to design your own HIFT workouts. Happy HIFTing!

THANK YOU

Rachel, Nicole, and Samir, you have been my confidants and my backbone since I can remember. My perseverance and strength came from having your shoulders to cry on. Kimberly, my dearest mother, although we had our differences when I was younger, you are now my best friend. Thank you for always being there on the other side of the phone when I need to talk. Bill, my number one dad, thank you for being wise and always guiding my way. Terralynn and Jordan, my sisters, your presence alone forces me to be a better and stronger human being. These few words don't even come close to expressing the love I have for all of you. Thank you for being you.

~ Ashly Hill

FIT WAY OF LIFE

FITNESS IS NOT A DESTINATION WITH

A FINISH LINE BUT A DAILY WAY OF LIFE

by Deirdre Slattery

Bachelor of Kinesiology, BKin
Bachelor of Education, B.ed,
Major in Primary Education (MPED),
Minor in Biology (MBio)
Personal Trainer, PT

Deirdre Slattery

Deirdre Slattery is a single mother of a beautiful daughter who is her greatest support and has brought out her passion to be her best — a healthy, positive, strong, and independent woman. She sees change as a constant opportunity to learn and grow from, and to make the best of life around her. She is an eternal optimist with a grounded and practical balance. This free spirit has spent time travelling the globe, learning about life, and feels most at home near water, with people living healthy and thriving lives, being happy and fulfilled. Helping others see their potential comes naturally to Deirdre. Her purpose is to inspire and motivate others to stay positive and strong through any adversity, as finding the good in every situation is what makes her life work meaningful.

Deirdre has a Bachelor of Kinesiology and Education from the University of Windsor with a major in biology and health education. She is following her heart after twenty years, to expand her career by educating and coaching others to live healthy and happy lives, and by helping them share tools to become the best version of themselves. Nutrition, exercise, and a healthy mindset are the foundations of her healthy lifestyle. Her future plans as an entrepreneur include making a greater impact in the health and fitness industry and lifestyle coaching. She feels most rewarded and fulfilled when helping others unlock and overcome their barriers to live the life they dream of. Deirdre has an open mind and heart, and is always there to provide a listening ear, or be a guide for someone looking to live a life of health, wellness, and happiness on a holistic level.

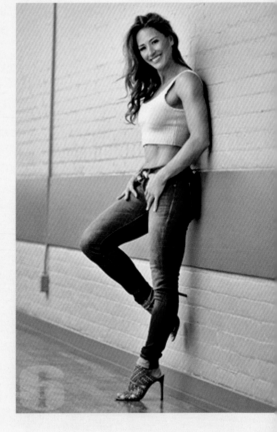

WWW.DEIRDRESLATTERY.ARBONNE.COM

Ig: deirdre_sfitness
Fb: Deirdre Slattery - Fitness and Health Transformation Coach

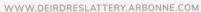

118

We often feel pressured to be on point in every area of our lives. The social mantras of *do more* and *be better* are louder than ever and it can be difficult to find a balance in which we are challenging ourselves and flourishing, while also remaining grounded and healthy. It's important to understand that it's not about being perfect, and doing *everything,* it's about striving to live an optimal life that works best for *you.*

As we understand that there is a positive relationship between physical exercise and self-esteem, cognitive function and achievement, this is a good place to focus if we want to live our best life! I've been passionate about living a healthy and active life for as long as I can remember, but one thing I had not done was push myself that last 5% to feel my best. I made the decision on my forty-fourth birthday to be the healthiest version of me I could be, to see what I was made of, and to improve my own self-esteem and mental health. What came from my personal journey was a new love for the gym, for eating properly to fuel my body, and to push myself to a new place of self-love, while helping to heal old wounds.

From my extensive experience in sports, strength training, bodybuilding, flexibility ,cardiovascular conditioning, personal training and wellness coaching, I hope to share some tips to inspire and guide you in your own unique journey. I will offer some tools to create a balanced fitness regime that suits you and your lifestyle best, no matter your age or stage of life. It's never too late to see what you're really made of!

Where To Begin (Pre-Workout)

What is calling you to start a fitness or gym routine? Maybe you want to feel better, have more energy, balance your hormones, emotions, and stress; maybe you want to look better, manage weight, meet new people; or maybe you simply want to try something different and take on a challenge! When we attach personal meaning to our fitness goal, we are more likely to follow through with it, even when the temptation to quit comes about, as it almost always does at one point or another.

We may feel social pressure to be in shape and have a perfect body, but external pressure can often be unhealthy and will not be enough to keep us motivated and inspired, let alone enjoy the process of getting fit and healthy. If we can find our *own* reasons, our own *WHY* on adopting a fitness routine, the time, discipline, and hard work will bear its own rewards as we achieve our goals and look forward to what's next!

So what is your *why*? Be specific and honest when answering this and write down your answer. Writing down fitness goals can make you 50% more likely to stay consistent and follow through with them and achieve success. The act of writing demands a deeper level of focus and clarity, while giving you direction in a world that is demanding you to go every way at the same time. What do *you* want? Write it down.

Here is a short checklist to get you started:

- Set a specific and realistic goal with a timeline
  What is your *why*? How will you achieve it? (i.e. what form of fitness/exercise best suits your desires and needs? What intensity will you start at?). When do you hope to see these results?
  Take before pics, chart how you are feeling, and take measurements. Check in on your improvements and changes every four to six weeks.

- Hire a trainer or join a challenge group for accountability. Get a gym buddy. Talk to your friends and family about your goals.

- What is the measurable part of your goal?
  We need to be able to measure success to know that it's happening. If your why is to have more energy, consider activities that you are too drained to take part in, but would like to. If your why is to manage stress and emotions, what are the circumstances or areas of your life that are negatively affected now, and how are they affected? What change would you like to see?
  Clues that you're achieving success are that you're feeling more rested, happier, it's easier to climb stairs, your complexion has improved, clothing is fitting better, you're lifting more sets, reps, and weight.

From Mind To Action (During The Workout)

By now, I hope your reasons to get healthy and fit are coming to the surface and maybe you are jotting down your big *why*. You are ready for your new way of living! We will only reach our goals if we act on our hopes and dreams. There is often a breakdown between *desire* and *doing* – life gets in the way and old habits are hard to break, but you can only begin new, healthier habits by taking action and implementing them, so get those sneakers on and start moving into a better you!

Here is an overview of the workout so that you feel confident and knowledgeable as you begin—the pre-workout, during the workout, and post-workout:

Pre-workout to ready the body: This begins in the hours ahead of the workout by being rested, hydrated, and well nourished. At the workout, we need to ready the body's systems with a proper warm up to get blood flow and oxygen to the muscles.

During the workout: We need to maintain hydration and proper breathing to ensure our body has what it needs to work hard. Take water breaks and learn proper breathing techniques for the exercise you're engaging in. This is also the time to individualize your workout and decide what best suits your needs. The options are endless—HIIT, interval training, yoga, aerobic dancing; what will help you to achieve your *why?* In order to achieve success, prioritize injury prevention with proper exercise techniques and progression, making sure you have proper guidance and knowledge during your workout.

Post-workout: We need to rehydrate, refuel, and cool down properly by stretching. A post-workout protein shake is a quick and healthy way to replenish and provide the muscle-repairing nutrients the body needs after its hard work. There are whey or vegan protein options — you will need to decide what is best for your body. Remember it's important to take rest days in your schedule, allowing your body time to repair and come back to the next workout ready.

Common Excuses (Post-Workout)

It's easy to start a new exercise routine when you're excited about making a change. The difficulty often comes after your first few workouts, when you realize you have to maintain these new healthy habits. Here are some common excuses to watch out for when it comes to continuing toward your goal:

Time: Life gets busy, so you will need to consciously make time with a daily method of operation. Schedule your physical activity as a priority and non-negotiable. Creating a schedule and sticking to it builds accountability and integrity in your word to yourself. Here's a tip: get your meal prep for the week done on the weekend to open more time for your fitness routine!

Tired: Beginning a new routine can be hard. If you're feeling tired from a busy schedule, exercise can seem overwhelming, but eventually each workout will leave you more energized, refreshed, and excited. Studies show that regular exercise acts directly on the central nervous system to reduce fatigue and increase energy, so stick with it! Here's a tip: have your gym clothes and gym bag ready in your car! When we arrive home from a long day it can be harder to be motivated to get back out again.

Money: The best investment you can make is in yourself and your health. Highly successful people incorporate fitness! Regular exercise helps the hippocampus part of your brain grow, which is linked to memory and learning—crucial skills for success. Exercise also strengthens connections in your gray matter, which is key in learning and even fighting off depression. So make sure you're remembering your *why* and are prioritizing your fitness goals. Different seasons of life bring different financial constraints, and there is plenty of exercise that can be done at home or outside for free! Jogging, free-weight resistance training, and yoga are all good options to do at home.

> The best investment you can make is in yourself and your health.

Guilt: Time away from the family, pets or work! When you make time for yourself, you come back to your commitments a better and more relaxed person! When you make health a priority, you set yourself up to be able to take on new opportunities for your family or work, as you will begin to have more energy and feel-good endorphins pushing you forward!

Insecurities: Some people feel as though they don't know what they're doing when they're at the gym or in a new fitness environment. That's okay! The only way to learn is to do, so hire a trainer or coach, get a gym buddy, have knowledgeable people to guide you and encourage you safely and effectively to build up your confidence! For an affordable approach, start in a group fitness class, or find a fitness video with great reviews to learn proper form. Here's a tip: visualizing yourself reaching your fitness goals can push you through moments of fear or uncertainty. Imagine what you want and shoot for it!

Hormones: If you feel as though you are constantly lacking energy, experiencing mood swings, or having heavy, painful cycles, you may have a hormone imbalance, as many women do. Exercise helps balance hormones and lessen symptoms of heavy periods.[1] Exercising can alleviate PMS symptoms by increasing circulation.[2] Yoga lowers blood-cortisol levels and releases brain-calming gamma-aminobutyric acid (GABA). Cardio increases dopamine and serotonin levels, and increases blood flow to the brain, which will elevate mood and decrease feelings of anxiety and depression. Work with your body and incorporate a workout or series of workouts that will aid in balancing your hormones while helping you get fit.

Diet: If you're not sure what or when to eat, see a nutritionist or hire a certified nutrition coach. Diet routines, just like exercise routines, are unique to an individual's needs. Make sure you are fueling your body properly to give you the best shot at success!

Extra Facts, Tips, And Tricks

Regardless of what your individual *why* is, here are some benefits of incorporating a regular fitness program into your life: developing a productive work ethic, working at a higher IQ level, improved sleep, decreased chronic pain symptoms, rehabilitating injuries, improving sport performance, decreasing risk of heart disease and diabetes, increasing longevity, improving overall life satisfaction and happiness, building self-confidence, improving muscle tone definition, skin complexion, sex drive, and more energy to do other things you enjoy!

Here's a list of nutrients that can help you reach your goals:

Magnesium: A key nutrient that helps metabolize estrogen. A buildup of estrogen can cause PMS, headaches, anxiety, depression, mood swings, or difficulty losing stomach weight.

Vitamin B: This helps to convert the foods we eat into fuel for the body, and helps to maintain energy throughout the day. Vitamin B can be found in all four food groups, including fish, poultry, eggs, and dairy.

Probiotics: a healthy gut is a healthy body! The immune system is largely found in the gut, so a daily probiotic can help to fight off sickness and keep energy levels up.

Vitamin D: The power of the sun can help to prevent osteoporosis, chronic pain, restless sleep, muscle cramps, fatigue, and weight gain. Supplement with vitamin D drops or spray if you are finding you have a lack of natural sun exposure.

Bromelain: A nutrient found in pineapple, which helps the body breakdown and burn fat.

Chromium Picolinate: A few studies suggest that taking chromium combined with a resistance-training program might help you lose weight and body fat while increasing lean body mass. It is used to treat type 2 diabetes (speak with a doctor if using insulin) and promotes weight loss. [3,4] Chromium is found naturally in cinnamon.

Healthy fats: Consumption of healthy fats decrease the risk of heart disease and stroke, reduce symptoms of depression, joint pain, arthritis, and skin ailments. Helps to increase weight loss, fertility, and energy. Adding healthy fats into your daily diet can be as easy as including foods such as avocados, wild salmon, eggs, nuts, chia and flax seeds, hemp hearts, dark leafy greens, and oils, such as olive or walnut.

If your *why* is to lose weight, whether it's for health reasons or a boost in energy and self-confidence, here are some tips and facts to help you out!

- Healthy body fat for women in your body mass index (BMI) is 17–25%
A good percentage to shoot for would be 20% unless you have more competitive or sport-based goals, keeping in mind that everybody is different, so be aware of how you feel.
- Excessive cardio isn't the way to lose fat—this is a misconception! The classic treadmill frequent flyer may have initial success with weight loss and changes in body composition, but after that, levels off and they may not see any more changes Incorporating resistance training into your exercise routine will help to convert unhealthy fat into muscle, and when you build muscle, it burns fat for you! Exercise post oxygen consumption (EPOC) is the body burning fat for 16–36 hours post-exercise! This will vary, depending on the type and intensity of the exercise, foods consumed pre-and-post workout, and the current state of health and fitness.
Many women are afraid of lifting weights because they don't want to look "bulky," but toning and building muscle is key in weight management.
Yoga, Pilates, circuit training, and resistance training with your own body weight (i.e. planks, crunches, and push-ups) are all forms of resistance training that will tone and tighten your body.

Here are 10 ways to burn fat and maintain your physical health for life:

1. Get moving: Consider additional ways to incorporate more movement into your life. Walk or bike instead of taking the car, take the stairs instead of the elevator, if you work a desk job, take small breaks to stand and help your systems to start up again, take time to play, whether it's with your kids or by yourself!

2. Chemistry (see chapter 3): Your body is a scientific machine with many systems that need to run properly! To get your body into the fat-burning zone, paired with the right levels of vitamins and minerals, aerobic exercise will increase your heart rate, get oxygen to muscles, and burn the fat! Make sure you are getting the following vitamins and minerals: magnesium, bromelain, chromium, vitamin B, and vitamin D.

3. Spice up your life: Ginseng, cayenne pepper, cinnamon, black pepper, mustard, turmeric, and ginger are just a few spices that help with weight management, so consider adding them into to your foods!

4. Water is life: Your body is made up of 60% water and every system in your body needs water to function properly! Water also helps your body to burn calories, so is a cheap and easy way to maintain your weight goals. The amount of water one needs varies from person-to-person, but as a general rule, women should be drinking eight to nine glasses of water a day. This amount should be increased in warmer weather and when exercising.

5. HIIT: Alternating high-intensity exercise with brief rest periods can give you better results in less time! One easy example is jumping rope for ten to twenty seconds, followed by thirty seconds at a slower pace.

6. Slow down: Be conscious of your eating in order to digest well. Ensure that you're breathing while you eat, and try putting the fork down between bites to slow the pace.

7. Timing is everything: Having breakfast first thing in the morning will make you less likely to overeat later. Try eating five to six smaller meals every three to four hours to keep your metabolism working and ensure steady energy levels!

8. Sleep on it: Make sure you are getting the right amount of sleep every night. As a general rule, you should be sleeping seven to nine hours a night. Any less *or* more can create health problems, which include weight gain.

9. R and R: Rest and relaxation is separate from sleep, and just as important. Taking time to rest with your eyes closed and your feet up can calm your mind, give your neurons a break, and help your muscles to recover, which will lead to a more productive life. Resting, or meditating, can help to reduce stress, improve mood, increase concentration and mental alertness!

10. A balanced life is a happy life: Be good to yourself! Remember that you can't do everything all the time. Having balance in your life is one of the healthiest things you can do for yourself, so refrain from going overboard on things, even if it's a healthy thing. A balanced diet, physical activity routine, and rest routine means allowing yourself a break when you need it.

I've learned from my own journey that your *why* will change as you evolve and grow. Embrace those changes and what you learn about your body and mind. Celebrate your successes and be patient and kind with your setbacks. Keep going and you'll get there!

THANK YOU

When we embark on anything new and daunting, it's good to recruit a team of friends, experts, and allies to get you on the right track, with outside support and knowledge. I would like to thank and acknowledge all the love and support I have received along my fitness and health journey, and a special thank you to my patient daughter Lily, my family, and friends. We can accomplish so much more when we work to push and support one another to achieve our goals and dreams.

~ Deirdre Slattery

YOU DON'T GET THE ASS YOU WANT BY SITTING ON IT

SMALL CHANGES DAILY, CREATE MASSIVE RESULTS OVER TIME. MOVEMENT IS MEDICINE FOR YOUR BODY AND SOUL

by Paula Man

Certified Personal Trainer, C.P.T.N

Paula Man

Paula Man has her diploma in fitness and health promotion, is a certified personal trainer, certified LeBert Equalizer trainer, and an accountability coach. She is a passionate warrior for helping women feel empowered, something which came about through many sequences of blessed opportunities. Paula has been featured on the tv show *York Region LIVE* for fitness & lifestyle segments, as well as radio talk shows for guidance on making fitness "fit" into all lifestyles for any person. She specializes in motivation, accountability, and empowerment. She strives to show her clients how strong they are and how they can reach their goals and are worth spending the time on to achieve.

Paula is an entrepreneur through and through. She owns her own personal training studio called Performance Fitness and she is also a proud network marketer. In both businesses, she uses her passion for leading through service and courage to allow others to step into their greatness.

Paula is wife to an incredibly sexy husband, Nick, and a mother to four beautiful little girls: Abbigail, Payton, Hailey, and Isabella. Paula understands the "I'm too tired," or "I'm too busy," reasons so many women have for not exercising. Her passion lies in showing women that it doesn't take hours and hours of super intense exercise that will have you not walking properly for days to see results. You can reach your goals and you *will* be successful, but you need to decide that you are *worth* it. The question isn't *can* you, it's *will* you?

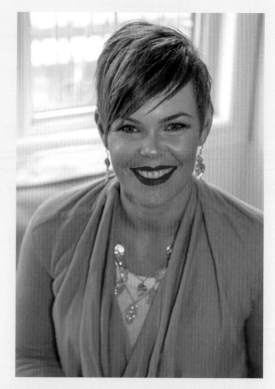

WWW.PERFORMANCEFITNESSTRAINING.COM

ig: paula_performace_fit | fb: paula.man.7

Have you tried all the latest workout trends, stuck with some of them for two to six weeks, been super excited about how you felt, then life happened and you fell off the wagon? Or have you done the workout your friend did and she got amazing results, but it did nothing for you? Or do you just not have time to exercise for 60-90 minutes, six times per week, like the "gorgeous people" do? Well congratulations, I'm here to tell you that you are normal!

My name is Paula Man, I am a mom of four little girls (all born within five and a half years... and NO TWINS!), I am the owner of Performance Fitness, and I have also been working as a personal trainer for fifteen years. Believe me, I understand the "no time," "too tired," "stressed," and "too expensive," barriers we all face as women in today's society. But how it that working out for us? We are in competition more than ever for the best mom award, most beautiful professional award, or just the woman who "looks" like she's got the perfect life, but is falling apart at the seams and feels like a failure when she's behind closed doors award. I personally felt that as a woman I needed to set some boundaries in my life in order to make myself a priority. Professionally, I started focusing more on how I could work with women to help them — through exercise. By helping them in this manner, I was able to guide them towards making themselves and their health a priority, so that they felt better physically, which then translated into more focus and clarity in their homes and business lives. Additionally, it also made them feel proud of what they were capable of and how strong of a person they were, which further enhanced their self-confidence.

My goal is to give you some useful information on *what* exercise does in your body and *how* to make exercise fit effectively into your busy life. I also want you to understand that you are *worth* your own time and focus, because you will be a better woman, wife, mom, boss, co-worker, and just happier overall. Lastly, I want you to give yourself a break and not beat yourself up for where you are now and what you haven't done in the past, but to look forward and realize that today is a new day and the only thing you can change is the future, not the past.

What Does Exercise Do For Us Physically?

Most of us know that exercise is good for us and that we should all be doing it, but I'd like to reiterate the list of benefits again just to show the magnitude of things it impacts internally for us:

- Reduces body fat
- Oxygenates the body
- Increases lifespan
- Improves immune system
- Improves memory
- Strengthen muscles and bones

- Help maintain mobility
- Manages chronic pain
- Reduces risk of diabetes
- Strengthens heart
- Clears arteries
- Lowers blood pressure
- Decreases stress
- Increase growth hormone
- Lower blood cortisol
- Reduce adrenaline
- Stimulate calming effects in the brain with gamma-aminobutyric acid (GABA)

The above list comprises all those things that we know happens inside our body, but we can't see it. Usually the goals we have are superficial, and we gauge them by things such as weight, clothing size, and measurements. The first thing you will feel when starting a workout routine will be increased energy — this can happen within a week.

Additionally, if you also clean up your diet by eliminating processed foods and sugars, and incorporate drinking two to three liters of water a day, you could lose quite a few pounds in a week or two. This can all be very motivating for someone at first, but when you head into weeks three and four, and you are still doing the same exercise routine, eating the same meal plan, but have reduced only one or two pounds, and you are tired and sore, it can be tough to stay on track. I found that even though I am a personal trainer, I wasn't getting my own workouts in, and it was because life

It's ok, I am a strong woman who is about to get her life, libido, and love for herself back.

was happening all around me and getting really busy with a growing studio along with growing kids. I had lost any "ME" time that I used to have. I was catching colds and flus, feeling run down, sleeping less, becoming more stressed, and because of all that, I chose to eat crappy foods, on top of no exercise! It's a vicious cycle, and I know I'm not the only woman on that hamster wheel. Are you nodding your head "yes" right now? I'd like to stop right here and have you repeat after me: "It's ok, I am a strong woman who is about to get her life, libido, and love for herself back." Now, grit your teeth and mean it! I am a strong believer in having positive thought patterns to combat all the negative thoughts we have daily. Your life follows the direction of your thoughts. So now that you have turned that corner and said out loud that you know you haven't failed at all and that you are about to become a badass woman on a mission, let's get a plan in place to help you do that. Exercise is a form of therapy and a reward for our bodies, yet so many of us see it as a punishment and work.

Exercise for us women can be an incredible tool to manage so many hormonal things we have happening on a daily basis in our bodies. There is research to show the positive impact exercise has on decreasing our signs of depression and anxiety as well as reduced chances for post-menopausal women to develop breast cancer.[1] As you can see, exercise is VERY POWERFUL! Most of the time people think exercise has a superficial meaning associated with it, but you need to understand that when you make a decision to put on your workout clothes and running shoes when you don't want to, or when you push those extra few reps when it's really hard, you are creating powerful shifts physically, internally, mentally, and emotionally. Be proud of the body you have as women; it's complicated, but when we lead a healthy lifestyle it can empower us do absolutely incredible things.

It is hard work, no doubt, but it is also nourishing and rewarding as the benefits outweigh any perceived limitations. It is easier to stay consistent with your exercise habits and enjoy exercising when you choose workouts that make you come alive, put a smile on your face, and forget about the burn in your muscles as you perform those movements. When you force yourself to perform a workout you do not enjoy, it will never become a healthy habit for you. Exercises such as Zumba or pole dancing are fun and amazing forms of exercise, or playing a sport you love is great too. Swimming or Nordic pole walking are amazing full body workouts as well. Crossfit and bootcamp classes are a few client favorites as these workouts challenge people to push their limits. All of these are forms of exercise: which one calls to you? If you want to experience and see results, the most important thing you need to remember is that you *must* be increasing your heart rate and keeping it up for a minimum of 20-30 minutes. If that is happening, then go crazy with whatever form of movement floats your boat!

Let's get into the finer details and choices that need to be made to set yourself up for success in the fitness game. We are going to go through and breakdown what I guide people on all the time in my accountability coaching sessions, bootcamps, and private personal training sessions: the *how-to* of getting results faster and in less time.

How Long Should You Workout?

I get asked all the time and most people's concept of workout time requirements are completely wrong! The mindset of "more is better" is what actually puts many people into an overstressed body that holds onto weight. Ideally, you want to schedule at least 30-45 minutes, four times per week, a fifth workout is okay too, but you also need to recognize that rest days are very important for your body to recover and rebuild stronger. Our society is flooded with the "do more, rest less" mentality, and it is literally breaking us down and aging us from the inside out. Rest days don't mean that you don't engage in physical activity, it just means that you do light activity instead of something intense. You can go for a hike or bike ride with the family, explore some trails, take a yoga class, or go for a walk with a friend or two.

The daily recommendations for exercise is 30-60 minutes, five times a week, so get moving most days. The great part about this is, even if you have to break it up into three 10 minute segments, it still has almost the same health benefits on your body. What I have seen over and over in my seventeen years in the fitness industry is that exercising three days per week for 60-90 minutes has LESS results than five or six days a week of heart-rate raising, sweat breaking exercise for 30 minutes each day. Why would that happen? Why would exercising more often for a shorter time frame produce more results? Well, if you know you have to only exercise for a short period of time, you are more likely to work harder during that time frame, compared to basically prolonging your energy for 60-90 minutes so that you can last. Secondly, you are more likely to stick to the routine because it's not a huge time commitment. Lastly, a habit has now been created where, if and when you do miss days, you actually crave the endorphins and the positive feelings experienced after your workouts. So remember, exercising 30-45 minutes, four to five times per week will create more results.

When Is The Best Time To Workout?

Here is the bottom line: The best time to workout is a time where you know you will do it consistently with little to no interruptions. So for example, if you find that 7:00 p.m. works better for your schedule, but then the kids have activities, or there is a work dinner that comes up, or you are tired from work, or any number of other things that can happen which lead to skipping your workouts more often than not, this is not a good time to schedule your workout. Another poor scheduling instance is if you want to workout before the work day starts, but you went to bed late the night before. As a result, you slept in, and are now unable to eat anything before your morning workout, since your time is limited. As a result, you do not push yourself to do an intense workout as you will likely vomit or faint due to hunger, exhaustion, and lack of sleep. This then, isn't a good time to workout either. What you need to do is be very realistic about your schedule and not what others tell you to do. In addition, no one knows your body like you do, so listen to it. Most of us know what time will work for us to workout, but we just don't *want* to do it so we use the excuse of "I can't fit it in." Listen to your intuition, it will tell you when it's time and don't overthink it, JUST DO IT! When you push yourself to take action, you won't always "feel" like it, *we never "feel" like it*, but decide that you are going to do this, no matter what, and DO IT. Once you have consistently made this a practice, you will then have created a habit for yourself which in turn will replace the old habit of talking yourself out of exercising.

You will need to carve out time, four days a week, for yourself if you haven't been in the habit of exercising regularly, but it *will* become a routine, and one that your body craves. Make sure you schedule your workouts into your week, just like you would schedule a meeting, lunch date, or kids' activity— it's non-negotiable.

Why Am I Not Seeing Results From My Workouts?

There can be many reasons for not seeing results such as not doing the right exercises, not working hard enough or frequently enough, not challenging your body enough to create change, or your nutrition hasn't improved so the workouts are pointless with all that you are putting into your mouth. So, let's walk through these together.

Not Doing The Right Exercises. To me, this is when people sit on a machine and focus on one body part at a time. The way I train my clients and what I always recommend to people is to do compound exercises or exercises that incorporate two or more muscles. When you do this, you make your workout really efficient because you use less time but work more muscles. In addition, you will also add a cardiovascular component to the workout instead of just strength training, and you will generally be doing movements that increase mobility through movements you perform on a daily basis.

You Are Working Hard Enough. I find that heart rate monitors are the best indicator for individuals to know if they are working hard enough during exercise — be it cardio or strength training. When you wear a heart rate monitor, you don't need to worry about lifting the same weights as the person beside you or doing as many repetitions, because if you are at 65-75% of your maximum heart rate, I promise you, you are creating some awesome changes in your body. A generalized calculation of your maximum heart rate is 220 – your age = maximum heart rate (For example, 220 – 37 = 183 maximum HR), then multiply that by 70% and 80% and you will have a range to work within (example: 183 x 70% = 128, 183 x 80% = 144 beats per minute). These ranges are guidelines, but rest assured that when you use these guidelines and try and keep yourself within the range of 70–80% of your maximum heart rate for the majority of your workout, you WILL see changes in your body. It is recommended that you should always consult with your doctor before starting any new workout routines.

Are You Eating For Results? Many people focus solely on caloric intake, however, I want to share my experience with you a bit here, and maybe guide you to reframe this dialogue, and think about the quality of your food rather that the calories it contains. Let's think about 500 calories. Do you think that 500 calories of a chocolate bar and a coke is equal to 500 calories of an apple with some natural peanut butter, and a few rice crackers? Of course not! Your body doesn't count calories, it recognizes real food, and it functions like it should with energy, aiding in muscle recovery, balancing hormone levels, and burning fat when it has the right fuel. [2] There is a popular saying, *"You can't out exercise a bad diet."* Eating well is a reward for our amazing bodies that do so many incredible things for us, *if we take care of them*, but so often, we reward ourselves for anything we accomplish with a diet rich in crappy, low vibrational, junk food, which drags us down on all levels. Feeling crappy isn't a reward. What you eat is so important in the discussion of results from your exercise routine.

How Long Will It Take To Create A New Exercise Routine? It takes anywhere from 21-66 days to create a new habit. [3] Everyone is different, but what is most important is that you focus on creating patterns in your schedule that work for you — for example, you carve out some time for exercise the exact same day & time each week. When you do that and stick to it for three months (90 days), you will start to crave it. Then, when you hit the 120 day mark, you will miss the feeling of being active if you don't do it. When you get to that point, you also will have created the ability to say no to other things because you have developed the habit of putting yourself first and self-care is important to you now. How does that sound? I'm telling you, it is a powerful and amazing feeling to have when you get there. No matter what form of exercise you've chosen, be protective of this time with yourself, it is sacred.

What Type Of Workout Is Best? Based on your personal fitness goals, there are many different workouts you can choose to incorporate into your exercise routine. If your goal is to gain a lot of muscle for something such as bodybuilding or figure competitions, you will need to do a lot of strength training and eat a lot! However, what I always encourage people to focus on first is making a consistent habit of exercising with a workout that incorporates full body, strength, core, and cardio. Once you start seeing results from these exercises, you can reassess your personal goals and tweak them more in four to six months if you aren't quite heading in the direction you want. When you focus on 30-45 minute workouts that get your heart rate up, exhaust your muscles, and challenge your core, you will lose inches, gain energy, and be *very* motivated.
Here is an example of a 30 minute workout that I would do with a client at my studio:
   • 5 min warm up (bike, elliptical, walking, stairs)

- Circuit as quickly as you can by getting through 3 rounds doing 30 seconds of each exercise listed below:
  - Circuit #1: Squat jumps, mountain climbers, bicycle abs, high knees
  - Circuit #2: Bent-over row, forward lunges with bicep curls, drop squats, plank
  - Circuit #3: Side plank, superman (for lower back), other side plank
- Stretch

Of course, there will be modifications for people with knee restrictions, etc., BUT you can see the workout style, and how efficient it can be. Best of all, it can be specific and personalized to each individual. No matter if you are just starting out or are a seasoned fitness buff, the goal is to move through each circuit as fast as YOU can, not comparing yourself to anybody else.

Another favorite form of exercise for me is Tabata, named after a Japanese scientist, Dr. Izumi Tabata, who studied at the National Institute of Fitness and Sport in Tokyo. What Dr. Tabata found was that 4 minutes of high intensity exercise was equal to or better than 20 minutes of moderate steady exercise. Both study groups experienced the benefits in aerobic capacity, but the high intensity group experienced much more improvement aerobically and also a benefit anaerobically. So you take any exercise and repeat 8 rounds of 20 seconds of work followed by 10 seconds of rest. There are many ways to combine or alter Tabata workouts to suit any person, but a true Tabata is 1 exercise, such as push ups done until ALL OUT exertion for 20 seconds, then total rest for 10 seconds, and repeat that cycle 8 times. As you can imagine, that would completely exhaust you. That can be done with any exercise, and you can get in 4 exercises in just over 20 minutes and have an incredible workout. For further reading on high intensity interval training (HIIT) and high intensity functional training (HIFT) exercises, and of course, some really good exercise sequences, definitely see chapter 8, written by my co-author, Ashly Hill.

Now GO DO IT!

No more over analyzing it, no more excuses, no more allowing yourself to feel exhausted, depressed, unmotivated, unworthy, and not beautiful! The line needs to be drawn in the sand and a decision needs to be made. You have the tools, the tips, and the information you need to set your plan in place for this week and get going on your journey. Will you step out and do it? I think, "what if…" statements are very powerful and I think they fit so well at this point for many: *What if* you started setting aside 20 minutes, four times per week for yourself to exercise each week? *What if* you could feel more energized? *What if* you could decrease your stress levels so you don't need to be on high blood pressure medications? *What if* you could be more patient with your kids? *What if* you could be an example to your kids and others — that living healthy can be done, even with a busy life? *What if* you felt like *you* again, instead of living inside a shell of you? Do you think it's worth it now to make yourself a priority?

> "I'm not telling you it's going to be easy... I'm telling you it's going to be worth it." ~ UNKNOWN

I'm challenging you to give yourself twelve weeks of focusing on consistent activity that challenges your heart rate and uses your whole body each time you exercise. I also challenge you to honor your body with what you feed it, remember food is your fuel, you need to feed it quality nutrients in order for it to do what you are asking it to do daily. I promise you, your body will thrive on movement and wholesome nourishment!

My hope is that you are fired up to get started on the goals you have for yourself that have been put on the back burner for too long. My hope is that that you will respect and honor the body you have been given and allow it to thrive, and for you to feel amazing again. It will take time and effort.

THANK YOU

Thank you to God who created me with a clear path and a fire in my belly to serve others with the gifts He has blessed me with.

To the love of my life, Nick, you are my rock, and I would not be the woman I am today without you standing by my side, holding my hand, and sometimes pushing me forward through every step of our journey. You are my biggest supporter through all my adventures and you have an incredible way of making me laugh each and every day as well as making me feel like the most beautiful woman in the world. I love you lots and lots.

And to my four gorgeous daughters, you are all such unique gifts to daddy and I. I pray that you are proud of your mama, but that you also see a strong woman going after her dreams, serving others with her gifts and always standing for what she believes is right. You all have special gifts that you have been given and it is an absolute blessing for daddy and I to watch you find those gifts and grow into them. Mama loves you so much.

And to you, my dear reader, for investing in yourself by reading this book; you are incredible, you are worthy, you are beautiful, and you deserve a life of abundance in all forms. I pray that this book will empower you, challenge you, and equip you to step into your power as a woman. You are reading this for a reason, so knowing that, use what you have learned to become the next best version of yourself. I believe in you.

~ Paula Man

CAKE, PILLS, AND A WHOLE LOTTA WEIGHTS

WHAT SORT OF EXAMPLE WAS I TO MY DAUGHTERS? I WOULD NEVER WANT TO TEACH THEM THAT ANY PART OF THEM WAS LESS IMPORTANT OR UNWORTHY, SO WHY WAS I TREATING MYSELF THIS WAY?

by Neli Tavares Hession

Certified Holistic Wellness Practitioner
Certified Holistic Nutritionist
Reiki Level 1 Certified
Certified Spiritual Life Coach

Neli Tavares Hession

Neli Tavares Hession is a mind, body, and spirit wellness coach and founder of MamaZen Coaching. She is a board certified holistic wellness practitioner with a concentration in holistic nutrition from Southwest Institute of Healing Arts as well as a holistic life coach from the University of Wellness. She is a reiki level I practitioner and Barbell Project ambassador through Gorgo Magazine.

She started her journey in 2007 after having frustrating experiences with traditional medicinal options for her then five-year-old daughter. Her passion is to bring the trinity of her services to empower women and girls to be their whole self and to challenge cultural norms surrounding the accepted values around women's bodies. As a client, you can expect to reconnect with your body through the mindful decluttering of anger, harmful affirmations and bad habits. She will help create a nutrition plan that will become both intuitive and clean, starting where you are at nutritionally. These meal plans will incorporate both a flexible diet with attention to macronutrients and balanced eating in the real world. Her mantra is to ditch the diet mentality and live a fit and healthy life without obsession.

Neli is married and lives on Rhode Island with her four children. She enjoys meditation, fitness, nature, and new experiences. When she isn't busy being a mom and running girls' empowerment workshops, she can be found working for her clients at

Nelihession.com, as well as on Facebook and Instagram.

WWW.NELIHESSION.COM
ig: neli_hession | b: neli.hession

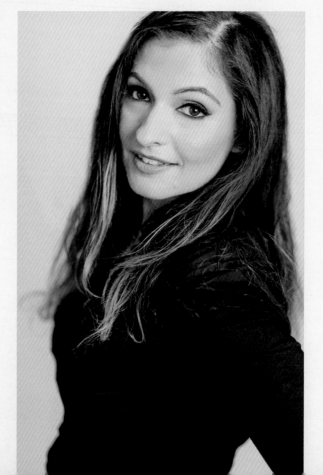

When I was a little girl, I idolized Wonder Woman, Superman, Popeye, and ThunderCats. Not only did I idolize them, I wanted to BE them. Watching Wonder Woman bust through doors and lift cars with nothing but her bare hands exuding this primal strength really spoke to me. I would go play outside and try to lift my parent's parked cars in our driveway, determined and *knowing* that one day I would surely get one to go over my head. Every day, I was on a different mission — be it to lift a car, a television, or a refrigerator, because to me, that epitomized power, strength, and courage.

As I grew older, my love of food took more precedence over any sort of movement. By the age of nine, I weighed 130 pounds while the average nine year old weighs 62 pounds. I was barely five feet tall, and trust me when I tell you, those 130 pounds were not all muscle. I would binge eat entire packages of Hoodsie cups followed by a whole box of granola bars. I would stay up late at night baking cakes and eating the entire thing alone— in one sitting. In no time, I was getting teased and bullied for my weight. My mother would encourage me to eat fruit because it was healthier. I did, but I would pour granulated sugar all over it before consuming it. My breakfast on most days would typically consist of several donuts and coffee (we're Portuguese, coffee is a huge staple in our diet, and we start young).

It wasn't until I was thirteen-years-old that I had my first dance with the diet industry. It was after a two week hospital stay for double pneumonia. I had caught a cold around Christmas time and refused to be seen by my pediatrician; my stubbornness landed me in the hospital. Staying in the hospital that long with no twenty-four hour access to my cake and ice cream obsession made the weight melt right off my adolescent frame.

Friends at school would comment on the new "skinnier" version of me and at age thirteen, that's all a girl needs: positive feedback on her looks. This was well before the "likes" and selfies of the social media world today. It was great. It was like a high. The attention was addicting. I wanted more.

Not being formally educated on nutrition or diet and not having any adult role models around that were well versed in this area, I did what any girl would do. I scoured the pages of *CosmoGirl* and *Seventeen* magazine and those commercials that came on TV after the soap operas were finished. That seemed like a legit place to turn to. All the pretty and polished women were representing me. Or *at least* representing what I *should* be.

I quickly learned that things like Slim Fast, Lean Cuisine, and tons of cardio seemed to be the go to way to get a new lean body. That's what they were all touting. And I bought into it hook, line, and sinker. Magazines and TV don't lie. Right? It took a good solid year to get the weight down to where I felt like I looked close enough to what I was seeing in those magazines and commercials. 90 pounds. I got myself to 90 pounds by the age of fourteen and it seemed like a good number because it wasn't triple digits. *Oh naive teenage mentality.*

Next stop? MODELING. Yep. I decided now that I was as skinny as those models on the magazines, I wanted to BE one of them. Thanks to my wonderfully supportive parents who raised me to believe in myself, I didn't think twice about this venture and neither did they. They took me to modeling agencies and photo shoots for composition cards. I was all in and so were they, *God bless their patient and understanding hearts.* Oh, did I mention I was only five feet and three inches tall? Yeah. Can't make it far in modeling if you're a short stack. But it didn't stop me. I wasn't going for runway. I was going for print ads, you know, those magazines that had gotten me started at the age of thirteen? Funny how things come full circle in some ways.

Anyway, there I *was,* determined to make it big in the industry, but whenever an agent would look at my composition cards and photos they would say, "You're beautiful. Striking. BUT... just not the look we are going for." I was told I didn't have that classic look that was so popular in the 90s. Women like Claudia Schiffer and Cindy Crawford were all the rage back then and there I was, a short Portuguese girl with curves. So I did what any feisty Portuguese girl would do. Gave the modeling industry the middle finger and took to weight lifting. Somehow in my head that seemed like perfect retaliation. Even back then, I wanted to be a trailblazer; #bethechange was always MY thing before it became a thing on Instagram.

At age seventeen, I had purchased my very first barbell set with my very own money. That was a huge deal. At the same time, I also fell in love with kickboxing. Both the lifting and the boxing made me feel so alive and empowered. It reconnected me to my childhood superhero self. I was hooked. That feeling of being untouchable and tough wasn't new to me, but this was on a whole new level.

Having just graduated school and having nothing more to do besides a part-time nanny job, left me with loads of time to myself. So instead of hanging around getting into trouble, I worked out. A lot. There would be days I'd work out for eight hours. I'd go to kickboxing in the morning for an hour, go to the gym to lift and do more cardio, come home and lift and do more cardio... and on and on until I felt satisfied. It was an obsession. An addiction. A seemingly healthy thing to be occupied with, but internally it was an unhealthy preoccupation. On "rest days," I'd feel restless and cranky. I swear I could feel my thighs spread because I wasn't doing much of anything. I would be crawling out of my skin because I wasn't working out. I would keep a log of all the workouts I did for the day and the duration and compare days. At that time, I had no idea about exercise addiction and eating disorders. Although I was far from a healthy eater at that time in my life, I may have purposely punished my body with exercise when I felt my eating was more out of control that day. It was my sister, who was maybe twelve-years-old at the time, who mentioned something about me possibly having a bit of an obsession with the whole thing. I brushed it off initially, because she's my younger sister and really, what does she know about adult things, but it did make me take a second look at how I was treating my body and living my life. My little social worker of a sister always seemed to have a knack for these things, even at the age of twelve. I had kept a logbook of all the workouts I was doing, when I was doing them, and how long these workouts lasted. I sat and looked back through pages and pages of so much intense activity, so many hours of doing nothing more than running, lifting, and kickboxing — no mention of me actually "enjoying" my day. Looking at those pages with a more discerning eye, I couldn't believe it. My days were truly consumed with exercise and not much else.

Things continued on a much lighter and more fun pace for a while after that. I had always enjoyed exercise, so naturally that was going to remain a part of my lifestyle, but just not on an obsessive level like it had been and I had finally come to grips with it. I'm forever thankful my little sister stepped in when she did.

At age twenty-two, I found myself pregnant with my first child. I was still very much physically active and continued to be very involved in kickboxing up until I was eight months pregnant. It was a running joke with my family how someone so pregnant could be throwing punches, kicking, and working out all the time. But I wore that like a badge of honor. I did make sure I kept it at a healthy level, checking in with my OB and getting her thumbs up the whole way through. Being pregnant forced me to come "home" to my body. Up until this point, there was a disconnection from it, oftentimes treating it like it was the enemy. Once I became pregnant, it was a different story. This was someone else's home as well, and I really wanted to do the best for my baby.

When my first baby girl was born, the weight came off easily. I'm sure being as active as I was helped that quite a bit. But still at this point, nutrition wasn't a factor of concern or worth a second thought. There would be days I would go the whole day without eating and then dry heave from feeling so ill from being malnourished. As a young first time mom, I didn't know of the "put your oxygen mask on first" concept to parenting. The thought of taking care of myself properly on the inside never occurred to me. On the days that I would eat, it would be double cheese burgers downed with a milkshake and followed by a big heaping ice cream sundae for dessert. There were tons of days of massive consumption like this. But the weight stayed off somehow, so I was never concerned. Why would I? I looked good on the outside. What more could I ask for, right?

At age twenty-six, I found myself pregnant again with my second baby girl. This time around, I had less time to exercise as much, but thankfully my cravings swayed

141

me in the healthier direction, so yet again, I was a bit lucky with keeping a "hot bod" to some degree. It wasn't until four months after she was born that I realized the weight wasn't just magically falling off anymore. Faced with less time to exercise and less energy, I did what any desperate housewife would do—buy into gimmicky "As Seen On TV" weight loss supplements. This was a time where Ephedra was all the rage. These giant horse pills packed quite a wallop laced with loads of caffeine and Lord knows what else. Whatever the "what else" was—I didn't concern myself with too much. They worked. I had the energy to tackle two small children through many sleepless nights. And the added bonus, my frame shrunk smaller and smaller each week. It truly was like magic. I could eat copious amounts of greasy, chemical-laden foods with reckless abandon and instead of gaining a pound, I was losing them at incredible superhuman speed. People were commenting yet again, at how incredible I looked—especially for just having my second child. Ah, there's that badge of honor again. What a great feeling! Except internally, I wasn't feeling too great. My body ached all over. So bad, I swore I had fibromyalgia. It hurt to the slightest touch. My hair was thin and like straw, and after a while it started to fall out. I would have constant panic attacks. I'd go for my yearly check-up and my physician was baffled as to why my liver levels were so low. I dared never to mention to anyone I was taking these stupid pills. Nobody knew. Not even my husband. There were news reports coming out about people dying from taking these pills, and yet, I'd convince myself I was different. Those people weren't following the instructions on the package correctly. That's it. They were doing it all wrong. I was totally doing it right.

The last straw with this pill fetish was when I woke up one night clutching my chest. It felt like I was having a heart attack. As I shot up holding my chest, I envisioned my funeral. *My children by my side. A young mom gone, all for the sake of being thin. How awful. How STUPID! What sort of example was I to my daughters?* I would never want to teach them that any part of them was less important or unworthy, so why was I treating myself this way?

An appointment with my physician later on revealed that I was deficient in several essential vitamins. No wonder I felt so sick and was in so much pain. Who knew vitamins played such an important role in overall well-being? I sure as hell never gave a damn up until that point in my life. It was always about what I *looked* like. As long as I could advertise to others that I was fit and trim, I was happy. Not once did it occur to me that how I felt on the inside—fueling my body for longevity and vitality, was more important than my stupid dress size.

That trip to the doctor's office opened up a whole new world for me. It ignited a deep interest in nutrition. Any down time I had, I'd research and read up on all things nutrition. I learned what vitamins played a key role in addressing some of the ailments I had previously from neglecting my inner wellness for so long. It was all so interesting! And it was all the more exciting when I'd apply what I learned on myself and I could *feel* the difference. My body was finally ALIVE! I started to eat to feel good, rather than a way to fix my looks. In the past, I had so many stories in my head about my looks or about food, and as you have read, none of them served me well. I overate to comfort myself or because "I deserved it." I would under-eat to quiet the loud booming voice of guilt from eating too much. All in all, I wasn't *listening* to my body at all. All of my experiences contributed to a horrible disconnect between my mind and my body's needs. And it contributed to so many unhealthy outcomes in terms of my overall health.

Four years later, I became pregnant again. This time with a baby boy. Armed with so much nutritional knowledge, I applied everything I knew to this pregnancy. I fed my body with superfoods chock full of vitamins and minerals to support a growing tiny human. I read up on the best foods to eat to help the baby's brain growth and development. The only thing I didn't factor in was after the baby came. The lack of sleep and time yet again got the best of me. My health and mental wellness was put on the back burner so I could "just survive," barely being able to take care of all the tiny people in my ever growing household. Ultimately I ended up with hormone imbalances likely due to years of dieting abuse, over exercising, and putting my body through three pregnancies, and sideswiped by postpartum depression. What started out as anxieties over my baby's well being (in reality, he was fine, but in my head, I was so sure he wasn't. One of the first signs of postpartum depression, postpartum anxiety, and obsessive compulsive disorder (OCD), most women aren't made aware of), quickly spiraled into extreme bouts of anger and aggression toward my husband, many fits of sobbing in closets and closed bathrooms, and then the scary terrible thoughts of harming myself came crashing through. Luckily, the thoughts were jarring enough to me that they signaled I needed help. Because I personally did not want to take medication, given my previous diet pill addiction, I dove deeper into my wellness and nutrition studies to find a more natural way to heal myself through this. Coupled with intense counseling, meditation, and really getting serious about my nutrition and taking care of my body, I found the end of that dark tunnel, thankfully.

By the time I had my fourth child, I had received my degree in nutrition, and had a good grasp on my own internal food and body demons.

I rid my diet of all processed, prepackaged foods, refined sugar, meat, and dairy and really started from the ground up. After a few months, I found that my hormones were in line again. What once was an every other week heavy menstrual cycle—consisting of several cycles per month—was now down to one cycle and at a normal flow. Mood swings were also a thing of the past. I became pretty well-balanced as far as temperament and mood go. My hair that had been thin, sparse, and straw-like for so long, was once again vibrant, full and thick. I had *natural* all day energy with no need for caffeine whatsoever. And to top it all off, I had a positive outlook on things once more. The brain fog I had attributed to just being a busy mom of many was eradicated as well. It was a true miracle! Who knew all this was possible just by eliminating "junk" from my diet, and eating nutritious, wholesome, and nourishing foods?!

There was so much more freedom to this new way of eating as well! I didn't have to count calories or fuss over fat or carbs because everything was healthy, natural, and nourishing. Eating this way allowed me to fully listen to my body's cues. If I was hungry, I ate until I was satisfied. If I wasn't hungry, I didn't force myself to eat because it fell into some sort of whacky self-perpetuated window of opportunity. I wish I could have saved myself years of feeling chronic fatigue and pain. I wish that I didn't engage in negative self-talk, body hate, rules, restrictions, and I wish I never went through scary depression. But I'm thankful for that harrowing journey because I'm using it to help heal others and make huge transformations from the inside out.

Now, it might seem counterintuitive that I'm not going to offer a nutrition plan in this chapter. After all, that is what I do for a living. I'm not doing that here because I truly want you to feel connected to *your* body and make food choices that serve *you*. I can't do that for you. And an "eat this, not that" list won't do that for you

Trust that your body wants real wholesome food and the rest will come naturally.

either. I don't want to deny you of your own amazing wellness journey. I believe we all know for ourselves what foods provide great energy and light us up on the inside and what foods don't offer much for us. While there is nothing wrong with guiding principles on nutrition, I believe feeling good is the most effective long-term reason to choose our foods. Trust that your body wants real wholesome food and the rest will come naturally. Don't be afraid to listen and more importantly, don't feel afraid to simply trust.

Although, I mostly eat plant-based foods, I am also a sucker for chocolate cake and a mean ice cream sundae. If I'm taking my family out for a dinner date, you'd better believe I'm enjoying the dessert afterward with no feelings of guilt or shame.

How To Start Your Own Wellness Revolution

Work out because you love your body, not because you hate it. Find a form of movement that brings you joy and do it for just that: joy. Again, if it's something you look forward to and enjoy, you are more apt to do it and do it often.

Enjoy real, whole foods in abundance.

Count nutrients and colors on your plate, not calories or fat grams.

Allow your intuition to guide your food choices. Keep in mind, real hunger comes on gradually over a period of hours in your stomach. Emotional cravings are strong and sudden and sometimes cause a feeling of panic or urgency. Note that this feeling comes from your head and not your stomach. If you wait it out for 15 minutes, these cravings should subside.

You are worth it. Oftentimes as women, as mothers, we take care of everyone else's needs before our own. Be sure to take these important steps to self-care and be strict about it. If you think about it, brushing your teeth is a non-negotiable item on your to-do list. This is such a strange concept to us moms, I know. But hear me out on this, the more you make time for yourself, the more it becomes second nature. And believe it or not—this has a huge impact on how you eat. You are less likely to overeat or binge because your "center" is calmer and happier. When you are calm and happy, naturally your food choices become more purposeful and nourishing. Slow down and truly BE with your body.

While I know our journeys are different, I also know from years of talking with women about their bodies that much of our struggles are the same. It is my hope that by being honest about my story, you find some hope, courage, and support in unlocking your own transformational journey. Take it from me, the answer will never be in a pill, shake, tea, or cream.

My journey has helped me coach hundreds of women into ditching the diet mentality, and help them live fit and healthy lives without obsession. So many of us are obsessed with being thin, or curvy, or toned, and so on. My life goal is to help all women drop the labels and focus on feeling amazing every single day. If we just let our body be whatever size and shape it wants to be—as long as *we treat it WELL*, how amazing would that be? We all get so caught up in trying to change what is, we miss out on what is truly important.

Energy
Focus
Strength (inner and outer)
Vitality
Emotion

What if we focused on feeling all of that?! Can you imagine the freedom?

My journey has helped me focus on feeling good and let my body be where it wants to be. I know my body won't disappoint me, and I can promise you that if you treat your body well, it won't disappoint you either.

THANK YOU

This is dedicated to all of the women on this beautiful planet. May we reclaim the fierce love of the warrior and embody the wisdom of the goddess to bring balance and harmony in our minds, bodies and souls.

To my mother, Isabel, thank you for always showing me how to consistently embrace courage and infuse risks into daily life rather than strive for perfection. Had it not been for those bold, valuable lessons, I would have never taken the leap to write and share my ideas with the world.

And to Bean, had it not been for your young wisdom, my journey through wellness may not have had as positive of an ending. I am always grateful to have you by my side.

~Neli Tavares Hession

NURTURE HER PLATE

Featuring

Amy Rempel

Tania Jane Moraes-Vaz

Allison Marschean

Jenna Knight

GETTING MY MENSTRUAL CYCLE ON POINT

WHY DO WE ALWAYS NEED TO COVER UP SYMPTOMS?

WHAT ABOUT THE ROOT CAUSE?

by Amy Rempel

Advanced Sports & Nutritional Advisor
& Aromatherapy

Amy Rempel

Amy Rempel has her degree in Communication Studies and is a Certified Exercise Nutritional Advisor, a bestselling author and is an Aromatherapist.

She is a mother to Asia and Will and has a very supportive and loving husband Ben, who was ready and willing to drastically change his health with her. As a family, they have been her biggest cheerleaders! She is a well-versed entrepreneur with over fifteen years in the health food industry, with experience in sourcing ingredients, manufacturing, sales and marketing. Amy helps women take control of their health and their family's by providing accessible plant based medicine and easy to follow protocols. She also teaches and trains other women in starting a sustainable business and how to utilize essential oils to further their purpose or career. She has a passion to help others achieve success with health and wealth by offering training in business, networking and product knowledge. She also volunteers in her community with a local drama club, sponsor's two girls in third world countries, and is a monthly donor to The Hospital for Sick-Kids in Toronto. Amy believes in empowering women to be their best versions of themselves by practicing self-care which is something that she teaches her team and family. The quote she lives by is "Above all, love each other deeply" - Bible, 1 Peter 4:8, just be sure to include yourself in this as well.

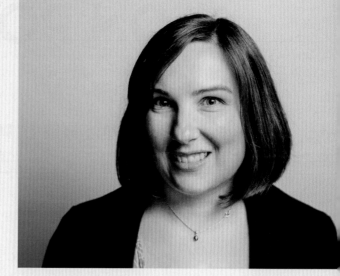

Connect with Amy at

rempel.amy@gmail.com or reach out to her on Facebook or Instagram.

ig: rempel.amy | fb: rempel.amy

The Beginning

When I first started getting my period at the ripe age of eleven, it was off to a rocky start. I missed at least one day of school per month because it hurt so bad. The main thing was the painful cramping. I barreled through each month like that until grade ten when I decided to go on birth control. At the time, although I didn't understand the havoc it would wreak on my body and that maybe, it wasn't a good idea to use synthetic hormones, it saved my life! My periods felt so much better and I hardly experienced pain or a heavy flow. However, I sometimes wonder if that ended up making things worse. According to Dr. Axe, birth control medications contain more than one type of female hormone. They're made with chemical hormones that mimic the effects of estrogen and progestin, which prevent pregnancy by stopping ovulation. [1] I continued to use birth control pills for ten years until I stopped doing so at the age of twenty-five, which was when I started getting leg cramps, making me feel worried about blood clots. These symptoms of a blood clot may feel similar to a pulled muscle or a "Charlie horse," but may differ in that the leg (or arm) may be swollen, slightly discolored, and warm.[2] These "Charlie horses" were waking me up in the middle of the night, I had enough! At this point I was married for a year, so I would welcome a pregnancy.

And Then I Got Into My Thirties

Eventually, we did have kids. I now have two children, and after giving birth to my second child at age thirty, my body shifted and then even more so by the time I was thirty-five-years-old. According to *Shape Magazine*, by age thirty-five, your fertility also starts to drop off and you may even begin entering early perimenopause, which can cause mood swings, sleep disturbances, and/or anxiety. Fibroids (benign uterine tumors) and endometriosis (a condition where the uterine lining migrates to other internal organs) are two conditions that are also more common at this age, and both can cause pain and heavy bleeding. [3] My menstrual cycle became unbearable, I was getting my period every three weeks and was always seven days early, which meant that sometimes I would have two in the same month! I would have premenstrual syndrome a week before getting my period, some of which included breast tenderness, cramping, and even occasional diarrhea (ugh!). The pain would ramp up the day of my period and my flow would be so heavy that I couldn't leave the house for about two days! I was too scared I would leak through or not get to a bathroom in time. The blood clots were so bad that I could feel them coming out and had to double up on iron every month so I wouldn't get dizzy from the blood loss. *It was nuts!*

I decided, since Western medicine was not able to help me without using synthetic hormones, to go to my naturopath and see how she could help me. Through diet and a supplement called DIM by Douglas Laboratories, my hormones and menstrual cycles would get regulated for about three to five months, but then go right back to how it was. The supplement was quite expensive too, so I would take it for about two months at a time and then take a break. This is actually how it's supposed to work, but eventually I would always have to get back on it. This was clearly not the answer. One thing I did know was that I had high estrogen levels, but I didn't know why.

Maybe Being A Vegetarian Is The Answer?

For a while, my husband and I talked about becoming vegetarians; we were doing meatless Mondays and sometimes an extra vegetarian day a week as well. But after watching a documentary about how going vegan or even vegetarian could help with various ailments, we started to seriously consider implementing it as a lifestyle change. My husband suffers from acute colitis and initially, this was the main reason for going off all mammal meat. Personally, I was more concerned about animal welfare as well as the environmental impact that eating meat has. According to the American Dietetic Association, appropriately planned vegetarian diets, including total vegetarian or vegan diets, are healthful, nutritionally adequate, and may provide health benefits in the prevention and treatment of certain diseases. [4] During this time, I also started a new supplement regime to help my joint health, hormones, immune system, and cellular health and discovered the incredible benefits of cypress oil (a therapeutic grade) for heavy flow and cramping due to menstruation. In fact, the leaf oil, when steam distilled, helps with "heavy periods, endometriosis and fibroids when applied topically." [4] That finding came from a friend of mine who said it had helped her fibroids (which had the same effects that I was having). Maybe I had fibroids this whole time? So as of August 6th, 2017, we stopped eating meat. On day one itself, my husband noticed he already felt better. He was digesting his food more easily and he didn't feel sluggish, so in turn had more energy. During the work week, for the very first time, he didn't experience the usual afternoon slump! Normally, he would have to work so hard at digesting his lunch that he would be sweating at this desk! I didn't notice a change until my dreaded period was due, except I couldn't tell when it was coming. I wasn't having symptoms as per my usual timeline and when I did get it, I was only four days early! Then the best part happened, in combination with using cypress oil I only had *one* small blood clot my entire menstrual cycle that month and I had ZERO pain! I kept forgetting I was on it! *What?!* I could not believe it. It was the miracle I had been waiting for! So, then what happened? I got a little lazy with my supplements and my daughter, who was not so happy about going vegetarian, wanted chili for her birthday dinner. "Real" chili, she stated. So, I thought, *what's the big deal? I'll eat meat once this month, there's no way it's going to impact me that much.* Oh my friends, did it ever. I had premenstrual syndrome (PMS) the very next day after eating beef chili! I ended up being ten days early! Thankfully, the cypress oil worked its magic and my cramping was bearable and there were no blood clots, but the week leading up to my cycle was terrible once again. I was convinced that whatever remedies I was implementing throughout August helped balanced my hormones, but of those, becoming a vegetarian is what had the biggest impact in balancing my hormone levels.

But I Buy Organic Meat!

I couldn't understand it, I was the mom buying organic chicken and grass fed beef—there's no added hormones in those. Then I realized I was using the word "added." Just because there were no *extra* hormones put in those animals, doesn't mean they don't have them. These are living mammals who breed, of course they have hormones; hormones that live in the body parts that we eat! As Dr. Michael Gregor has found, it's not a matter of injected hormones, which are banned in Europe in order to protect consumers' health. Sex steroid hormones are part of animal metabolism, so all food of animal origin have these hormones, which have been connected with several human health problems. [5] I am convinced that this had been the root of my problem. Undoubtedly meat is a valuable nutrient source for humans; there are however, increasing concerns about the safety of meat due to the excessive presence of steroid hormones. [6] Even animals who are raised properly and healthy contain those hormones and we add additional levels of them to our body, as a result of consuming meat products. Consuming a lot of red meat, ham, processed meats, soy products, or alcohol (especially beer) appear to increase the risk of developing fibroids. [7]

> Even animals who are raised properly and healthy contain those hormones...

Premenstrual Dysphoric Disorder (PMDD) Perhaps?

I also noticed that in the days leading up to my period and usually for the first day, I was always feeling very emotional. Things that I hadn't thought of in a long time would come into my head, or I felt sad for no reason at all. I definitely had mood swings, but I also had the blues. It is the strangest feeling because there was never an obvious reason for it. There was nothing that had happened in my life when this struck, except for PMS. Now, this is something else that has changed. My mood is *much* more stable and I'm even in a good mood! I no longer get down before or during my period. And this was me: Premenstrual dysphoric disorder (PMDD) is a more severe subtype of PMS that involves more types of emotional symptoms (such as sadness, anxiety, mood swings, irritability, and loss of interest in things). Women suffering from PMS-related depression and PMDD report dramatic relief from their symptoms once their menstrual flow is underway. [8] *Ain't that the truth!* The University of Copenhagen in Denmark has studied more than one million girls and women aged between fifteen and thirty-four over a thirteen year period. They found a very clear link between using the birth control pill and suffering depression. Adolescent girls using combined oral contraceptives had an 80% increased risk of antidepressant use and those using progesterone-only pills had a 120% higher risk of being on antidepressants. [9] Could this also be a side effect when off of birth control? I was on it for a long time and never had PMDD symptoms beforehand and it is a hormonal response. PMDD is tied to the hormonal changes triggered by ovulation, so it does not occur without this part of the menstrual cycle. Turning to a healthy diet, giving up cigarettes, and starting an exercise regimen are just a few things that can help. [10]

What's interesting is that as I have been researching I have learned so much more about myself and the different things that I probably have had but was never officially diagnosed with. I probably suffered from PMDD and fibroids, but I never looked into it further because I know so many other women who suffer with the exact same health concerns, so I figured it was normal. What was disturbing was that during my research, so many articles stated that a lot of these symptoms are "normal" and to "take over the counter meds" to help with those symptoms of PMS. Why do we always need to cover up symptoms? What about the root cause? Let's get rid of the problem that is causing these symptoms! I don't think these symptoms are normal and I now know there is a solution. Every woman is different, but if we can learn to understand our bodies and how it reacts to certain foods, exercise etc., then we can help it as I have seen in myself with multiple issues. I truly believe that our body is built to heal itself from ailments like PMS or PMDD through diet, essential oils, and proper supplementation.

Watch Those Stress Levels

I have read that stress levels can cause an influx of estrogen, so this is something I have tried to manage utilizing clary sage oil. Linalool, which is another key constituent in clary sage (*Salvia sclarea*), produces enzyme inducing and sedative properties, which would definitely explain the instant calming effect it has on me after inhaling it. [11] As a busy mom, this is very difficult. I seem to go in waves of busy-ness; sometimes I feel like it's under control and other times there is not enough time in the day. I'm sure many of you can relate! But we must learn to control stress— because when stressed, our bodies release cortisol, a hormone that may cause an estrogen imbalance and block the effects of testosterone. [12]

A Learning Experience

What I have learned is that we, as women, have so much more to be aware of. We need to learn about how our bodies work and to listen to them more often than not. We have the ability to utilize our intuition, which is something we can learn to use more efficiently, but that's a whole other chapter. If you feel something is not right and you have a diagnosis that seems impossible to heal through Western medicine, look into it further. Get second opinions, go to a naturopath or a traditional Chinese medicine (TCM) practitioner. There are other (and sometimes better) ways to help our health when we treat it naturally through diet, essential oils, and proper supplements. These are the ways in which we can help the root cause of a problem instead of just treating the symptoms. For so long, our health has been dictated by other people, but it doesn't mean we always have to take one diagnosis as the end result. We need to be the ones who have power over our own bodies and ways to treat ourselves.

> "At the end of the day, your health is your responsibility."
>
> ~ JILLIAN MICHAELS

THANK YOU

Thank you to my wonderful parents and ALL of my siblings for always supporting me and checking in with me, even when they weren't too sure about what I was doing. And of course, thank you to my biggest support system, my two awesome kids, Asia and Will and my amazing husband Ben. I love all y'all SO much!

~ Amy Rempel

EMPOWER AND HEAL YOUR BODY, MIND, AND SOUL WITH PURPOSE, PASSION, AND KINDNESS

"BEAUTIFUL GIRL, YOU WERE MEANT TO SURPASS MOUNTAINS. NOT THEIRS, BUT YOUR OWN."

by Tania Jane Moraes-Vaz

Tania Jane Moraes-Vaz

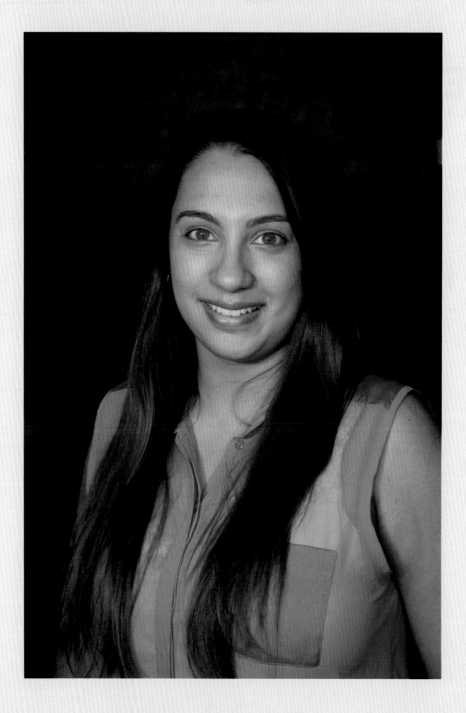

When asked to sum up her life mantra into a sentence, Tania truly feels that, "Passion always propels change, and kindness always heals everything." Armed with the principle, Tania believes one can certainly achieve all that they desire and live the life they have always dreamed of. A graduate from the University of Waterloo, with a B.A in English Language and Literature, Tania is tenacious, passionate, creative, eclectic, eternally optimistic, and highly intuitive—traits that have helped her persevere and grow, while empowering her to create momentous change for herself to lead a life of choice and design.

She is a mindset and empowerment coach for women with Polycystic Ovarian Syndrome (PCOS), lifestyle photographer, 2x best-selling author in *Dear Stress, I'm Breaking Up With You* and *Dear Limits, Get Out Of My Way* (editorial commentary), and overall creative maven. Tania enjoys living life to the fullest and capturing moments ("Carpe Diem" might as well be her middle name)—be it through the lens of her camera, blogging, or a notebook when she's on the go. These outlets have been her saving grace through life's challenges, as well as a medium for celebration.

Six years ago, when Tania was diagnosed with PCOS, she created a whole new lifestyle for herself built on a foundation of being passionate, positive, fierce, kind, and relentless about wanting change for oneself on a holistic level. Through her wellness journey, she noticed the sheer lack of awareness around women's hormonal health issues and realized her purpose and passion was to spread PCOS awareness by guiding and empowering women to live a holistic lifestyle through mindset and lifestyle changes. An avid learner and healer at heart, Tania always turns to nutrition, natural therapies, and energy work to manage her PCOS and alleviate her ailments. Her 2018-2019 studies include holistic nutrition, pranic energy healing, and neuro-linguistic programming (NLP).

Tania lives in incredible Mississauga, Ontario with her husband, Alan, and their adorable son, Arnold. Connect with her on the below platforms to learn more about her work, offerings, or even have a virtual chat over a cuppa herbal tea and yummy eats!

WWW.TANIAJANEMORAESVAZ.COM
Ig: taniajanemoraesvaz | fleetingmomentsbyjane
Fb: PCOSthrive | taniajanemoraesvaz

The Day My Life Changed Forever

I believe that we always remember the most important dates/events in our lives. They are life changing and are usually moments that alter the course of our life, leading us to examine who we are as people. They end up having a significant impact on us, and how we show up in our life thereafter.

For me, that date was none other than Friday, November 17th, 2012. Unknown to me in that moment or on that day, my life as I knew it would completely change. Everything I once knew to be safe or normal, no longer would be. It was a complete upheaval of everything that was status quo. An awakening. A rebirth or a second chance at life.

Around late afternoon at work that day, I started experiencing a sharp pain in my stomach, towards my lower left abdomen. At first, I didn't make much of this pain, as it kept coming in short bursts or spasms. I thought I had simply overworked myself the night before at the gym, so I kept to myself, worked away, and took frequent breaks to rest, thinking that maybe I ate something weird and was having a reaction to it. Eventually, the pain was so severe, that I couldn't sit straight in my chair without keeling over to the right to relieve the stabbing jolts of pain on my left side. I couldn't breathe properly and felt like enough was enough. I needed to go see a doctor.

I left work early and drove myself (*don't ask me how—God / the Universe was definitely watching over me in this condition*) to my family doctor to get checked. I couldn't even manage to walk properly, and as soon as she saw me enter her clinic, she gave me a requisition to go to the ER. I drove myself to the local hospital, simultaneously calling one of my best friends to let her know that there's something wrong with me. Next, I called my mom, and asked her to meet me directly at the ER.

I checked into the ER around 3:00 p.m. that afternoon, was seen by all the doctors on call, yet two hours later, none of them could determine what was wrong with me. They ruled out appendicitis and nobody could tell exactly *what* was causing this pain. Meanwhile, the pain was escalating constantly. I usually have a high threshold for pain, but about six hours into waiting in the ER, I broke down completely. I asked my mum to check and see if they could give me something to keep the pain at bay—morphine was my comfort for that moment.

This worked for about an hour or two, but eventually, the pain came back with a vengeance. By this time, it was around 11:00 p.m., and I was taken into a separate treatment room in the ER, where they kept prodding and checking me. I swear I felt like a lab experiment. If they had suspicions about what it was, they weren't telling us anything. Eventually, they got me over to the ultrasound centre for a pelvic ultrasound. This was the moment of truth.

They diagnosed a swollen and twisted left ovary and multiple enlarged cysts, which were the source of pain I had felt all day. Now I knew why I was unable to breathe properly. They let my mum know that I would need emergency surgery right away to drain the cysts and of course untwist my ovary, since it was graying in color and could also affect the right ovary, which could result in a complete removal of both ovaries. Around midnight, I was taken into emergency surgery. The last thing I recall the Ob-gyn saying was that they would do all that they can to ensure that everything is okay.

Lights out. It all goes dark.

November 18, 2012 - My "Very Common" PCOS Diagnosis

The next day, my Ob-gyn came to check up on me and of course discuss exactly what was happening within my body. He told me that I had a condition known as Polycystic Ovarian Syndrome (PCOS), and that it is very common among women: 1 in every 10 have PCOS.

He mentioned this can be managed with diet and lifestyle changes such as eating healthy, exercising, but also with medication such as the birth control pill (which I blatantly refused to go on, given the horrendous side effects it does carry, but that's a story for another time), Metformin, and other medication which would help my body get back to itself. I let him know I led an active lifestyle—I practiced yoga, went for walks and runs, and also worked out at the gym regularly, although my eating habits were still all over the place. He mentioned that in more cases than not, it's quite hard to actually lose weight with PCOS. It's typically a case of what came first: the weight or the health condition? Meanwhile, I think to myself, *Okay, this doesn't sound so bad. This is something I could handle. How hard can it be, right?*

Next, he lets me know that PCOS is one of the leading causes of infertility, so I might want to come see him whenever I decided to have children. He said that my chances of conceiving a child were 1 in 50, and the odds of not having a child, or not carrying a pregnancy to full term were a lot higher for someone with PCOS. And even if I did choose to go with IVF etc, my chances were slim to none, statistically speaking.

Cue blurriness, white noise, confusion, anger, not really listening anymore to anything he or anyone else is saying to me in that moment.

My thoughts were all over the place: *I am only twenty-three-years-old. I just graduated. I guess this is what it feels like when someone tells you that you most likely won't have kids. You didn't even know that you wanted kids, Tania. But wait, I have yet to meet the right person for me, to be able to build and grow a family with. I am so young. Why is my body working against me? I will overcome this naturally. I will take it upon myself to help myself, and things will be okay. I trust God / the Universe to help me in this.*

Although he initially recommended that I start taking birth control as a way to manage symptoms and regulate my menstrual cycle, I firmly let him know that I did not want to go on allopathic medicine, instead, I would work to reverse or at the very least, manage this naturally through various natural remedies and therapies—I didn't quite know what yet, but I'd research my options and keep him updated. He told me that everything would be okay, I just needed to go home and rest for the next two weeks, try not stress out too much, relax, eat healthy, and take it easy. He let me know that whatever I chose to do—whether it was to go on allopathic medicine, or alternative medicine—he would support my decision all the way (*bless his heart, honestly, the best Ob-gyn ever*).

Where there is a will, there is always a way. You just have to dig deep within yourself to find it, and follow through. So for the next two weeks post surgery, while I took time off to rest, recover, and process this newfound information and diagnosis, I started going gung-ho researching different naturopath clinics and looking for different ways to manage and thrive despite my PCOS diagnosis. Did you know that 1 in 8 North American couples struggle to conceive? Fifteen percent of North American couples are affected by fertility issues. If this is North America alone, you can only imagine what the statistics may be on a global scale. Infertility does not discriminate on race, religion, sexuality, and socio-economic status. [1]

Through my reflection, incessant curiosity, and mission to heal myself as holistically as possible, I realized that I might have always had PCOS, I just never *knew* I had it, and it definitely went undiagnosed until of course, I ended up in the ER at the age of twenty-three.

Flashbacks of my adolescent years took me down memory lane, and it all started making sense to me: having hair on my chin and neck (*this literally made my life a living hell through high school and university, cue the bullying, and the isolation, and of course never wanting to be around any members of the opposite sex)*; the constant weight fluctuation—no matter how hard or often I exercised; pretty much getting to a point of not eating anything in front of most relatives or family friends due to subtle and not so subtle body-shaming (I never seemed to "look" healthy or fit according to them); the summer in university where I had a crazy amount of skin tags but I thought I had some sort of weird rash or skin condition (I only discovered they were skin tags when I was diagnosed with PCOS); and of course the massive amount of anxiety, mood swings, and constantly feeling out of place from my own body because I could never figure out why my symptoms existed, or why my body never seemed to work with me.

PCOS - A Silent Epidemic With Its Own Complications

PCOS is a condition in which a woman's levels of the sex hormones estrogen and progesterone are out of balance. This leads to the growth of ovarian cysts (benign masses on the ovaries). PCOS can affect a woman's menstrual cycle, fertility, cardiac function, and physical appearance. According to the U.S. Department of Health and Human Services, between 1 in 10 and 1 in 20 women of childbearing age have PCOS. The condition currently affects up to 5 million women in the United States. [2,3]

PCOS Is Multifactorial – Stress, Lifestyle Factors, And Genetics

According to Hormone.org and Healthline.com, while the exact cause of PCOS is unknown, doctors believe that hormonal imbalances and genetics play a role. Women are more likely to develop PCOS if their mother or sister also has the condition. Overproduction of the hormone androgen may be another contributing factor. Androgen is a male sex hormone that women's bodies also produce. Women with PCOS often produce higher than normal levels of androgen. This can affect the development and release of eggs during ovulation. Excess insulin (a hormone that helps convert sugars and starches into energy) may cause high androgen levels. [2,3]

Symptoms Of PCOS

These usually vary from woman to woman, but the most common indicators and symptoms are listed below. [2,3]

- Irregular menstrual cycle
- Missing menstrual periods
- Issues with infertility
- Hirsutism – Excess or unwanted body or facial hair growth
- Weight gain and trouble losing weight
- Acne
- Skin tags
- Darkening skin
- Depression or anxiety
- Poor sleep
- Sleep apnea
- Pelvic pain

Some Complications Associated With PCOS

These usually vary from woman to woman, but the most common complications are listed below. [1,2]

- Infertility
- Diabetes, and insulin resistance (elevated levels of insulin)
- High blood pressure
- High cholesterol
- Anxiety and depression
- Sleep apnea
- Endometrial cancer
- Heart attacks
- Breast cancer
- Uterine cancer
- Ovarian cancer

Whew. That was quite a lot of information to come across, and of course, digest mentally and emotionally.

Did I really want to overcome this naturally and let my body heal itself with time? YES.

Was I ready to face this, and start my lifestyle and diet change right away? Uh, NO.

A large part of me knew that I needed to take the necessary steps to kickstart my healing process, but I was not yet ready to face it head on. My heart knew that I needed to make this change, my mind however, was nowhere close to accepting this. It had a mind of its own (pun intended).

Suffice it to say, 2012 ended with few more weekends of unhealthy binging on junk food, alcohol, and desserts. Ironically, or through fate, or Divine Providence, it was around this time (during my recovery post-surgery) that I met my significant other, Alan. Little did I realize or know at that time, that somehow fate / God / the Universe was working in my favor (recall, I mentioned my Ob-gyn telling me I needed to find my "one" soon and start trying for children when we were ready). I truly believed Alan to be the one for me right when I met him. We have been married for almost three years now. He was, and has been my support, my rock, my biggest cheerleader and advocate, and my toughest critic throughout my health and wellness journey.

Ripping Off The Bandaid

2013 started out with a resolve to tackle my health condition with persistence, kindness, and lots of effort and consistency. I had researched quite a bit about natural ways of treating PCOS, and decided to go see a naturopath to help make this a reality. This was how I came to see my naturopath and acupuncturist. My first appointment with them was almost two hours long. For the first time, I felt like someone understood what my body was going through, and I could make sense of quite a few things thanks to their guidance:

- *Why I was unable to lose even a little bit of weight, despite exercising consistently*
- *Why my body reacted the way it did, and wreaked havoc every time I ate out (restaurants, fast food, etc).*
- *Why I just couldn't stand the taste of dairy, but I kept having it.*
- *Why I felt like my stomach was always in knots, and looked like I was bloated beyond measure no matter how often I exercised.*
- *Why I constantly had issues falling asleep, and of course felt exhausted every single day. Even on days where I did manage to sleep through the entire night.*

By the end of my visit, my naturopath asked me a few questions that really resonated with me. The below questions ended up becoming my cornerstone for my daily decisions, choices, and of course eventually went on to influence my lifestyle and diet changes as well.

- *How am I managing my stress levels? What are the sources of my stress?*
- *Can I work on prioritizing myself first by eliminating my sources of stress on a gradual basis?*

She mentioned to me that going through this treatment protocol for PCOS would mean a complete lifestyle and diet change. And a key part of this change would be learning how to better manage my stress, as this played a huge factor in my hormones going out of whack. This protocol would be a complete change of direction. My healing would not happen overnight and would take anywhere from three to six months to start seeing results, and of course, over time and with consistent effort, I would experience a more permanent shift in my health, and get better.

That night, I accepted and acknowledged that *I did not gain this weight overnight.* I realized that my health did not get to a point of me needing emergency surgery overnight.

I did not suffer from chronic stress overnight. Rather, it was a steady progression from my childhood and the stress and trauma associated with it. It kept building up internally, until it manifested itself psychosomatically.

Through this realization came another—*my hormones did not decide to have a daily block party overnight.* Rather, this was a steady progression, and a culmination of genetics, nutrition, lifestyle choices, chronic stressors, and trauma. And guess what? This could be overcome.

I could change things for myself if I followed my protocol to a T to start with. And more importantly, *I could only accomplish this if I had the emotional and mental mindset to thrive and overcome this.*

I was to take natural, bioavailable supplements (fifteen different ones) two to three times a day for the next six months, and we would then revisit my protocol, and see what we could eliminate further, based on my progress. In addition to this medical protocol, I was to completely switch my diet to a wholesome, nutritious, non-processed one. I was to:

Eliminate all gluten, refined and processed carbohydrates, and foods. Stick to complex carbohydrates such as sweet potatoes, brown/wild rice, squash, fox millet, finger millet, and quinoa for sources of carbs instead.

Eliminate dairy. Switch to almond, rice, cashew, hemp, oat, or coconut milk instead (recall, I mentioned earlier that I have never been able to stand the taste of dairy my whole life, yet I kept having it. By eliminating dairy consumption, I learned that my body automatically knew what worked for or against it).

Eliminate alcohol completely. Alcohol wreaks hormonal havoc in our bodies due to the sugar content, especially when one of the major symptoms of PCOS is insulin resistance.

Eliminate refined sugars. Start using stevia, dates, coconut sugar, and honey to sweeten teas, or any foods if I craved a sweet taste. This was by far the hardest thing for me to eliminate (all those who know me, know that I have a huge sweet tooth!). Have dark chocolate (think 85–90% dark chocolate) as an alternative instead. Use cacao powder as a substitute for hot chocolate—mix it up in a hot cuppa dairy-free milk. Voila, you have your protein, magnesium, and iron fix right there, not to mention, soulful comfort in a cup.

Limit caffeine intake to 1 cup of tea or coffee a day, and eventually eliminate it completely. Consume more herbal teas such as peppermint, spearmint, ginger, ashwagandha, reishi and chaga mushrooms, and chamomile. Use Dandyblend as a coffee alternative, or if you must consume caffeine, try green tea or matcha tea instead —the benefits are phenomenal.

Eliminate or limit my intake of red meats, and poultry. Or find a clean protein source by buying organic, non-synthethic hormone injected, grass-fed meats as much as possible, if and when I chose to have meats as part of my diet.

Have lots of greens and vegetables. Follow an alkaline and plant-based diet for the most part, and have a clean and sustainable protein source—if I was ever having the hankering for some protein.

Have foods rich in healthy fats such as, avocados, nuts and seeds, hemp seeds, chia seeds, and other clean, sustainable protein sources.

Have fruits with skin such as kiwi, pears, papayas— a great source of fiber to bind toxins and excess estrogen and detox it naturally. Limit overall fruit intake to a few times a week, as these could still cause spikes in blood sugar.

Essentially, I had to reframe my perspective around the word "diet" with "nutrition." I decided to change my perspective on these so called eating "restrictions"—I saw this as a way to nourish and nurture myself internally and externally through wholesome nutrition.

In addition to the supplement and diet changes, I was given a series of self-care tips to implement that would result in a total lifestyle change over the years to come such as:

Castor oil pack therapy. Great for hormones, reducing ovarian cysts, detoxing, and relaxation. I was to apply this at least twice a week every week on my liver and lower abdomen area (excluding the menstrual cycle week). To this day, this therapy works wonders hormonally, physically, and mentally. It is one of my go-to remedies on any given stressful day or week.

Working out regularly, but this time, I would work with my body, and not against it. This meant more plyometric exercises, swimming, yoga, high intensity functional training (my co-author, Ashly Hill has some really great HIFT sequences in chapter 8) instead of long cardio sessions. This meant moving more in sync with my body, depending on how it felt on any given day. Some days, it would be dancing, or kickboxing. Other days it was just plyometrics and weights, and some other days, it would be yoga.

Getting more Zzzz's in. Learning to sleep more, and take more naps. Learning to disconnect from technology and people if I needed to.

Journaling regularly. This would help calm my monkey mind, and serve as a sounding board and reflection tool.

Meditating, praying, reflecting more so that I could calm my stress levels, and take a step back instead of my cortisol spiking chronic fight or flight response.

Taking relaxing baths using magnesium salts, and make essential oils my new BFF. Magnesium bath salts have detoxifying properties, and ease aching muscles and joints, aid in relaxation, nutrient absorption, and increasing insulin sensitivity. Essential oils such as lavender, peppermint, and clary sage are known for their relaxing and hormone balancing properties.

Using non-toxic cosmetics, skin care, bath and body products, and also home care cleaning products. I had already started dabbling into using more natural products in my time in university, but I wasn't completely there yet. Armed with my PCOS diagnosis, this was incentive to learn more and educate myself on product impact, the ingredients our skin and hair ingests, and their effect on hormonal health. Over the last few years, almost all my makeup, hair care, and skin care products are natural and vegan.

Most importantly, learning how to say NO to things that weren't Tania-friendly: alcohol, unhealthy habits, patterns, behaviors, toxic environments and relationships. Learning to be okay with putting myself, my health, my time and energy first, instead of constantly depleting my energy by overextending myself to everyone and everything. I could no longer function the way I had been functioning for so long— *Being "on" from 5am Monday all the way till 3am Sunday had to stop. No more long overcommitted weekdays and weekends. No more saying yes for the heck of it. If it didn't make me feel good, or wasn't good for my health, it had to go completely, or it had to be managed.*

Hmmm, did that sound like a tall order? I didn't think so. I was essentially asked to put wholesome, healthy, nourishing foods into my body, so that I can heal myself inside out. I was asked to take care of myself not just physically, but also emotionally and mentally. I had to pretty much unlearn everything that I thought was true and good for me, and re-learn how to cope, heal and thrive—especially in a socio-cultural environment, where for the most part, people were and are unaware and ignorant because these kinds of health conditions are very taboo topics of discussion.

I was asked to give myself the gift of holistic healing. This was definitely different and atypical of the norm in our society, and it still is. However, I believe that maintaining or regaining optimal health truly is a holistic process, it is never about any one aspect. I needed to address it holistically, in order to get to the root cause and heal myself.

I realized that, yes, my progress wouldn't look the same as someone else's. PCOS looks different on every woman. "Healthy" looks different on every woman. I was asked to respect my journey and be kind to myself during this process. I was asked to make myself a priority. A non-negotiable priority. For once, I decided I am going to do just that.

Heal Yourself Girl, You Got This!

What happened next? I said, *heal yourself girl, you got this.*
How? With love, persistence, faith, and the right support system (which includes yourself)

So, I set out to undo years worth of health damage—not just physically, but emotionally and mentally, and start my healing process. One step at a time. One day at a time. This was not an easy feat, and it still isn't on some days.

Over the last few years, I learned how to become better at saying NO, and putting myself, my health and well-being first. Was I always 100% consistent at doing this? Uh NO. Did it get easier to say no, and be good to myself as the years passed? YES.

In this process, I lost a few relationships, and gained some new ones. I lost some jobs, and had to walk away from some other roles, but ended up discovering exactly what my calling and my purpose was, met my wellness and business tribe, and stepped actively into being a source of

What happened next? I said, *heal yourself girl, you got this*.

empowerment and support not just to myself, but to other women who I knew were battling PCOS or something similar.

Was this a hard pill to swallow? YES. Letting go of toxic environments, habits, patterns, and people really does suck. But that is only because it is is all you have known, and as a result, you were used to the said dynamics within home and work environments, and respective relationships. You didn't realize or know that there was a different way to go about this. A way to actually be kind to yourself, put your-self first, which automatically aligns with your health needs. So, yes, in the mo-ments that these transitions were taking place, I never really understood them, I would question things. I would question the loss of jobs, friendships, and other re-lationships—*why is this all happening all at once?* It was a lot of change.

However, whenever I had some quiet time and thought about it, I accepted and acknowledged that this is all part and parcel of my healing process on a holistic level. I swapped a whole lotta negative for an unending barrel of positive. At least, I chose to see it that way. Having a fierce, positive, kind, and em-powering mindset was the biggest component to my healing process.

> ## Having a fierce, positive, kind, and empowering mindset was the biggest component to my healing process.

It wasn't always easy to say no to foods I couldn't eat, to always stick to my lifestyle and diet choices. It most definitely was not easy to do this in front of family, or even some friends. I hated having to explain my-self, or constantly say no. Some moments, I was plain weak, and lacked the resolve to stand up for myself, and of course binged out on high sugar and fully refined foods. Other times, I just stopped seeing family or if I saw them, I wouldn't eat in front of them. I'd eat ahead of time, so that I didn't get tempted at any events. But most of all, having the right support system around me helped me stick to my heal-ing process a lot more.

My family slowly came around and understood *why* I needed to eat a certain way, and do certain things. There was nothing cuter than when my mom told me,"*Tania, I have baked a gluten-free, sugar-free, and dairy-free cake for you. Not sure if it tastes good, but I'm starting to learn how to make foods you can eat too. I don't want you to feel left out for desserts. I will learn to make more foods that you can eat.*" Thankfully, Indian cooking has some great options for that, and I have experimented and cre-ated some really cool variations on traditional Indian dishes that I too can enjoy.

My best friends always planned our get together menus keeping me in mind, and always helped steer me back to my path of self-care, and were a huge source of strength and support. And my significant other was always supportive by spread-ing awareness and knowledge among his family and friends about what I could and could not eat, and they too were onboard with my health journey. He was my advocate when I was still learning to be strong for myself and put myself first. There were numerous occasions he would help me say no to things when I couldn't muster up the courage to do so (*think of social galas, dinner-dances, and numerous community gatherings and parties, where I would have to literally explain why I don't want to drink, or why I couldn't have something, or why I needed to leave at a certain time so I can get my much needed rest*). He would also support me by not eating or drinking foods that I couldn't have, when there were no other options at a public gathering, or just surprise me by either cooking or buying me foods I could eat. And yes, ladies, he still does this, to this day.

I realized that in addition to having a wonderful support system in my significant other, family, and best friends, *I* played a huge part in the quality of my own health and well-being as well. How? *Through my mindset. Through persistence.* Following my instincts by advocating and researching about my health condition incessantly—to the point where I pretty much only stuck to the "whole foods, reverse this naturally route" because I was scared, and sick and tired of feeling sick and tired. The alternative was never an option for me. It was a one track, tunnel vision mindset of "My body can heal itself, I can do this. I deserve to be healthy." I could either be my biggest cheerleader and push on towards progress, or I could sabotage myself, my growth, and my healing by letting doubts, negativity, unhealthy habits, patterns, and behaviors consume me all over again.

Pffft. Diet, And Lifestyle Changes - Does It Really Work?

Yes. It does. It does work, but it requires YOU to make it work. It's not easy; there will be days where you will feel tempted to simply go overboard and binge (I had a ton of those at first, and that is totally okay, don't beat yourself up about it), but slowly you get over it. Once you feel and notice the positive difference in how your body feels internally, you'll want to binge less, and strive for more balance— whatever you deem that balance to be. It may mean having a small bite of an amazing gluten/dairy/sugar free dessert instead of devouring it instantaneously. It might mean making homemade foods that you can eat, or purchasing a few treats that only you can eat. For some, it might mean going without any temptations in sight, so that they are able to adhere to their health protocol (I know I had that approach at the very get-go when I started for at least a good while). Now, I personally keep a handful of treats on hand for those few in between moments where I am craving something. This has helped me slowly get rid of my craving for refined sugary foods.

The "learning to say no" muscle only gets stronger as time goes by, because you will be exercising this muscle daily for your nutrition and lifestyle choices. I always believe that saying no paves the way for more heart and soul centered yes's. Eventually, it'll be an immediate internal response instead of second guessing yourself. You will be able to walk away from overcommitting, overextending, and overexerting yourself. Once you discover what it truly feels like to put your health first, all else in your life will align exactly with that, from the people you choose to associate and interact with, to the career path you choose. In some cases, you'll manage a stressful career path much better once you are mindful of your health, and you'll make lifestyle and diet choices that benefit you instead.

Fast forward a few years later, my significant other and I got married in 2015, and we decided we wanted to start trying to have our family. Given my journey with PCOS, we knew that we may have a tough road ahead of us, despite all the diet and lifestyle changes that I have made over the past few years. It was time to see if the lifestyle change, the nutrition overhaul, the putting myself first thing really did work. Was it possible to completely prep your body for pregnancy a few years prior? Yes. We were blessed with a cute little baby boy in August 2016. *I, who was told that I had a 1 in 50 chance of getting pregnant naturally, and if I did want to get pregnant, I'd have to go the IVF route (which also has a slim success rate statistically for women with PCOS), was able to conceive and carry to full term, a healthy baby boy.* I was shocked, and could not believe this. And this was when I realized that your body is a miracle waiting for you to tune into it. Your body has the power to create life, and it definitely has the power to heal itself. Being able to conceive naturally made me realize that with a persistent, nurturing, kind, focused mindset and relentless faith and action, purposeful miracles are very much possible. This was mine.

When I initially found out we were pregnant, I was pretty much shocked, surprised, and overjoyed. I couldn't for the life of me believe that my body had ultimately worked with me and made this possible. Deep down I had thoughts of *I knew it was possible, I just didn't believe that it was possible for me.* Crazy, right? Not really, especially when all you constantly face from people around you is negativity and ignorance towards your health condition, and all you are surrounded by are the infertility statistics of women with hormonal disorders, and the naysayers. Although PCOS symptoms vary from woman to woman, it doesn't mean that they can never get pregnant, it just means that women with PCOS are at a higher risk of infertility given the risk factors and complications associated with it. For me, the work doesn't stop here, it is a total lifestyle change for me on a holistic level which has become a consistent habit, and is now the cornerstone of my day-to-day life. Eventually, we hope to slowly have newer additions to our growing family.

I understand that this is a really sensitive topic, and respect that each of us have our own journey with health and wellness. I am not here to judge yours, nor can I even fathom what you or your loved one may be going through. I am here to simply share my journey and spread more awareness in hopes that it inspires even just one person, and provides a personal perspective to someone who may be battling similar health concerns. Remember, you are not your diagnosis. Whether or not a pregnancy is the result of your nutrition and lifestyle change, several things are certain — you will change and grow for the better, and will learn to set better boundaries in your life so that all toxic influences are limited or eliminated. You will learn how to love yourself more, how to thrive and really use your talents and share your purpose with the world.

Know that you have it within you to create positive, long lasting change for yourself, everything else that comes from it is a bonus—an effect caused by the daily actions and choices you make. Please be gentle with yourself, and kind to yourself, no matter what your health circumstances, and no matter what the end result is. Love your body: learn to understand it, and be attuned to it. Your body has the power to heal itself, but will only do so when you learn to understand it and work with it, both emotionally and mentally. Advocate for it. Be your own savior and cheerleader first. And most of all, have faith. Unrelenting, undying faith in yourself, and your body. You are a masterpiece; your body is a temple —give yourself the time you need to heal yourself holistically. It is all possible. One day at a time. One choice at a time.

THANK YOU

I'd like to first thank my Lord, Jesus, for the gift of my life; for blessing me with the gift of motherhood and for our darling baby boy, Arnold. You have always been my strength and guide, through all the storms in my life. I will forever trust in your mercy, love, grace, and divine providence.

To my husband, Alan, you are my rock and my post. Thank you for supporting me in the ways that I "need" instead of want, for honoring my multi-passionate and free spirited soul, and for being an amazing hubby and father. You have been a crucial part of my health journey and healing. It may often go unsaid, but I love you more than you realize, and I'm grateful for our life together. I cannot wait for the rest of it to unfold.

To my darling baby Arnold, you are my my biggest blessing. I love you. You gave me back my true self, and your brave soul has taught me to fight for my dreams and the life that we deserve—fiercely and fearlessly. You have taught me to choose grace and kindness over perfection. Mummy loves you Arnie boy!

To my mom, thank you for nurturing my dreams and always being there for me, and now my family. You have shown me that unconditional love and kindness heals everything.

To my best friends, thank you for your unconditional love, acceptance, and support. For making me laugh, wiping my tears, celebrating my wins, and being my family.

To my mum-in-law Ana, for welcoming & embracing all of me—quirkiness, mood swings, bear hugs, protecting me like my own mum, and for always thinking of my health and well-being and doing whatever it takes to make things effortless for me.

To my naturopath and acupuncturist (Dr. Lara), my Ob-gyn (Dr. Tigert), thank you for supporting me wholeheartedly on my wellness journey, and showing me our bodies really are meant to work with us, for us.

To Ky-Lee Hanson, for being my angel in disguise from the time I met you. I am so thankful I said YES to writing with you two years ago. You are not just my publisher and colleague, but are one of my best friends, an older sis, and one of my biggest #bossbabe inspirations. Thank you for all that you do. And most of all, thank you for creating and nurturing a space where I am able to express myself freely and fiercely, and for making quite a few of my dreams come true already. Thank you for believing in me and always seeing the best in me.

~ Tania Jane Moraes-Vaz

ALLOW YOUR BODY TO HEAL FROM THE INSIDE OUT

WITHOUT QUESTION, WE CONTROL OUR ATTITUDES OF MIND AND HOW WE NOURISH OUR BODIES!

by Allison Marschean

Allison Marschean

Allison is a wife to Vince Marschean and the mother of three girls—seven-year-old twins, Brynn and Piper, and a thirteen-month-old Jordan. She majored in French at The United States Military Academy at West Point, NY and graduated in 2001 with a Bachelor of Science in systems engineering. Allison also holds a Master of Science in management of technology from Murray State University and a Master of Arts in organizational psychology from Columbia University's Teachers College. Currently, she serves as an officer in the United States Army Reserves and has a combined total of seventeen years in both the Active Army and Reserve Components.

A true believer in the healing power of food, Allison has put plant-based eating to the test more than once. Each time, she experienced healing as a result.

WWW.ALLISONMARSCHEAN.COM | WWW.HELO4U.INFO
ig: allison_marschean | fb: allison.marschean
li: allison-marschean-b22988108

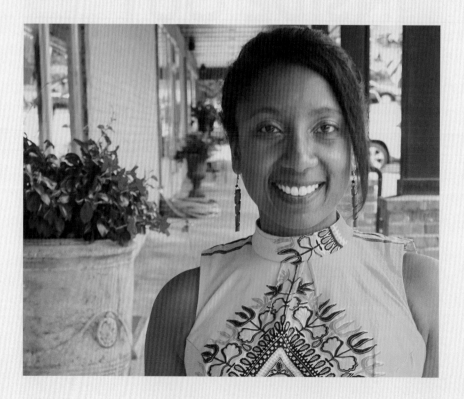

Years ago, a marker was planted along my journey. This came into my life by means of a plaque at a keepsake store. It helped me put things into perspective, and encouraged Vince and I during our challenging journey toward parenthood. If I knew then what I know now, I would have been fully content with God's timing and his entire plan for that difficult time in our lives. Very easy to say after the fact, I know. But let me tell you, EVERYTHING about his timing was, and is, perfect!

Our story began the summer of 2007, when I became pregnant soon after our honeymoon. I was twenty-nine and my husband was thirty-seven. We didn't want to wait too long to start our family, so we were eager to get started! Unfortunately, we had a miscarriage in August 2007, when I was roughly five weeks along. What a physically and emotionally painful experience that was! Aside from the pain, the hardest part was that we were stationed at a post where there were families who were expecting a baby, or who had just had their baby. As a dual military couple, my husband and I were fortunate enough to be assigned to positions that granted us the flexibility to make frequent trips to our reproductive endocrinologist (RE). More importantly, my boss was extremely sympathetic to our situation and supported my morning absences from the office. I cannot think of any other Army assignment I've had where this would have been possible!

It took some time for us to become comfortable with trying to conceive again. I didn't know if I could take another loss. Part of me was scared to try for fear of a similar outcome. In fact, I was having such vivid dreams of bleeding again that I would wake up in the middle of the night to check. My husband, of course, didn't want to see me in the excruciating physical pain that I was in with the first miscarriage. Time passed, my body healed, and anxiously, as we held our breath, we tried again, and were pregnant soon enough. I remember attending a baby shower, and one of the guests joyfully announced that she was pregnant and moving into her second trimester. I really wanted to spill the beans, but I knew I had to wait one more week. This time I was one week away from completing the first trimester. And yet again, that opportunity did not come. Before the week was over, we made another trip to the ER. The physical pain was more intense this time, probably because I was further along than our previous pregnancy. It didn't help that the two young soldiers triaging me were drenched in cologne, hence making me feel even more sick! As they pushed me in a wheelchair to the exam room I told them, "Someone's cologne is making me feel sick." Surprised, they mumbled something and both tried to take credit for the offense. April 2008: a second miscarriage, another heartbreak, loss, confusion, and pain marker in our journey of parenthood.

Sadly, the military hospital would not send me for further testing because "having a couple of miscarriages before a successful pregnancy is not uncommon." So basically, we'd have to suffer a third loss before anyone would be overly concerned. On November 9, 2008, we had another positive pregnancy test and by December 4, not even a month later, we were back in the ER. Of course, I did what I did the previous two times and racked my brain to figure out what I'd done wrong. *I must have messed something up. Was it because I would take two stairs at a time at work or was it the coffee table I helped to lift?* I searched for causes blaming myself for each failed outcome. In fact, by the second miscarriage, I had convinced myself that pregnancy was a fragile process—one wrong move would destroy the life inside of me. The ER routine was unfortunately becoming what we expected, but that is exactly what it took for doctors to examine our situation more closely.

After three miscarriages between August 2007 and December 2008, our obstetrician decided to test our blood for something she had not encountered in her nineteen years of practice. On December 22, 2008, with a house full of family for the holidays, my husband and I exited the house a little anxious and a little excited for our 9:30 a.m. appointment. What would the doctor tell us? Would we be her first case in nineteen years or would the news be less complicated and shocking than that?

Alas, we were her first case in nineteen years. While all of my tests came back negative, my husband's came back positive for a balanced translocation. We learned that he does not have run of the mill DNA. Essentially, he has the standard number of chromosomes (46), however, when he was conceived, his number 1 and 13 chromosomes (1p:13Q) switched places. This swapping of genetic material makes it difficult to reproduce—it sounds extremely dismal when you are not familiar with how far science has come in this area of study. We later learned that there is such a thing called an unbalanced translocation which is the more complex of the two and makes the conception of a healthy child, or any child, much more difficult.

Balanced or unbalanced, at that point it was all the same to me—we weren't going to be able to have children—at least not our own biological ones. Upon hearing the news, I felt hopeless and wanted to cry. I even felt like I was going to pass out right there in the doctor's office. Since I am big on taking notes I forced myself to stay focused and capture everything the doctor shared to ensure we knew exactly what the way ahead looked like. At the same time, I was thinking of my husband who must have been really hurt to hear the news. For forty years of his life, he had no idea that he had a genetic condition that could affect his fertility. We left the doctor's office a bit hurt, a bit angry, but mostly just feeling shocked.

When we got home, all I wanted to do was be by myself in my room and cry, which is pretty much what I did. My husband on the other hand, is a problem solver. He immediately began researching scholarly journals online to see how to overcome this balanced translocation. As we suffered for the next several days, I could not help but feel bad for my younger sister who was roughly three months pregnant. She must have felt horrible knowing that she was having a successful pregnancy while we had just been given some pretty devastating news.

We were referred to a geneticist and by the time we had our first appointment on January 13, 2009 *(interesting that the date matched the balanced translocation nomenclature 1/13)*, thanks to my husband's research, we already knew mostly everything the geneticist shared with us. Our next step was to get a referral to a reproductive endocrinologist (RE) and our first appointment was on February 13, 2009. *Funny, how all of our appointments kept taking place on the 13th!*

Our in-vitro fertilization (IVF) journey was not a hole-in-one experience. While our RE and his team were phenomenal, it was a lengthy process. It took us so long to achieve success that one of the nurses said that we were the longest running patients the clinic ever had. Due to the balanced translocation, we had to send all of our embryos for preimplantation genetic diagnosis (PGD) to ensure that they did not have genetic problems that could lead to additional miscarriages.

Our first IVF cycle produced thirteen embryos *(there's that number again!)*, but only one embryo passed genetic testing. That embryo was transferred, but did not implant successfully. The second cycle of stimulation produced plenty of eggs, but threw my hormone levels completely out of whack. My doctor advised against a transfer because he could tell from the lab work that an embryo would not survive. He suggested that an Endometrial Functions Test (EFT) be performed to determine the state of my uterine lining. The EFT established that my uterine lining had too much protein, making it officially dysfunctional.

Rather than try to conduct a transfer directly after a cycle of stimulation, my doctor advised that we wait a bit and do another round of simulation. The plan was to retrieve as many eggs as possible in order to create embryos that could then be sent for pre-genetic diagnosis (PGD) testing all at once. After two rounds of simulation we accumulated and froze twenty embryos. Of those, four survived the thaw and PGD. The next step was to get my uterine lining ready to tolerate a transfer. For several weeks my husband gave me intramuscular progesterone injections every night (in my rear end). At the same time, I was also taking three endometrin vaginal progesterone inserts daily.

On February 17, 2011 two of the four hardy embryos were born. After three years of setbacks, our little girls, Brynn Liana and Piper Romae, entered the world! They are more amazing than we could have ever dreamed! Brynn's middle name is a form of Eliana, meaning "the Lord answers our prayers." She is very animated, daring, has big brown eyes, and a playful grin. Piper is an observer with an infectious giggle, who does things at her own pace, and whose two massive dimples melt hearts. They are constant reminders that life truly is a miracle.

In the end, I could see that God's timing for us was perfect on all fronts—personally, financially, and professionally. He set everything up from the start! Even before we knew what lay ahead, He was working to put us right

where we needed to be. From being accepted to our graduate school program in New York to the casual, oh by the way, referral to Dr. Michael Blotner and his exceptional team, looking back, everything was right on time. Military insurance does not cover the cost for IVF because it's viewed as experimental, but we were able to afford the cost because of our dual-military income. Had we conceived and become parents when WE wanted to, we wouldn't have been able to devote as much time to our jobs as we did.

On August 24th 2016, our two remaining embryos were thawed and transferred. One implanted successfully and Jordan Elizabeth was born in May 2017. Having Brynn, Piper, and Jordan in our lives is worth all of the heartache and pain we experienced along the way. Remember the marker that was planted in my journey by means of a plaque? Well, that plaque now hangs in my home and it reads, *"Life isn't about waiting for the storms to pass, it's about learning to dance in the rain."*

4 Activities Of Encouragement When Overcoming Fertility Challenges

Keep a journal. Journaling can be very therapeutic and is an excellent way to capture all the feelings and emotions *(trust me, there will be many)* you'll experience along the way. One of my journal entries chronicles the first night my husband and I struggled to prepare the medicine. I wrote: "Wow! It just took us two hours to prepare and inject my dosage of Menopur and Gonal!! We started at 1800 hours and it is now a little after 2000 hours. We watched the DVD for a refresher but couldn't figure out how much diluent to reconstitute the Menopur vials with…" Of course, preparing the medications eventually became second nature, but I'm glad that I captured those moments in my black and white composition book! One day we'll share these stories with our girls!

Put your thoughts in check. It is very easy to get discouraged by failed attempts and setbacks. After a while with no success, I wanted to throw in the towel. I was physically and emotionally tired. I played the "what if" game. Focusing on questions like "What if this doesn't work again?" isn't helpful. There *is* power in our thoughts! William Shakespeare said, *"Nothing is good or bad, but thinking makes it so."* Zig Ziglar also offers sound advice concerning our thoughts, *"You cannot tailor-make the* *situations in life, but you can tailor make the attitudes to fit those situations."* Regardless of the outcome, make every effort to go through the process with optimism and cast aside all anger, bitterness, and doubt.

Choose hope. For us, it was either do IVF and PGD for however long it took achieve success **or** suffer more painful miscarriages. Considering our options, IVF gave us the most hope. What gives you the most hope? Hebrews 6:19 (NIV) says that hope is an anchor for the soul. [1] Make the decision to anchor your soul in hope. Find something about your situation that offers even the tiniest bit of hope, and cling to it!

Visit an acupuncturist. My RE recommended I visit an acupuncturist and tell said acupuncturist that I needed to increase the blood flow to my uterus. I located a phenomenal acupuncturist, in Middletown, New York. He was pleasantly surprised that a Western medicine physician highly recommended that I receive acupuncture to increase the likelihood that an embryo would successfully implant into my uterine wall. Believe it or not, it was the embryo transfer after the acupuncture treatments that was successful.

5 Things You Should Know Before Beginning IVF Treatments

The underlying cause for the inability to conceive or keep a pregnancy. There are a number of reasons a couple may have difficulty conceiving or experience miscarriages. The key is determining the root cause. Keep in mind that it could be the male input to the equation. Determining the principal cause will dictate the remedy.

Cost. How do you plan to finance your efforts? Knowing what your insurance will cover and what you will have to pay out of pocket is huge! Also consider how long your finances will allow you to fund your efforts.

Your reproductive endocrinologist. Be sure to do your homework. Questions to consider include: is your endocrinologist and his/her team well respected? What is his/her practice like? What are the success rates for that practice? Reading reviews will certainly help you make an informed decision.

Your contingency plan. What's your backup plan? What will you do if you're unsuccessful the first time? Will you try again? Will you adopt a child, look for a surrogate, or seek out an egg or sperm donor? Knowing your next move will help you better accept a failed outcome even if the next move is not the most desired one. There are more people than you realize who struggle. Most people struggling with fertility tend to keep their fertility journey to themselves. But it's important to know that more people struggle to have a baby than you realize. Although you might think you are alone, you are not alone. There is strength in collectively sharing each other's journeys, learning from one another, and being a source of support for one another.. Find that support system, and know that you are not alone in this. Thinking back on those times in my life, I feel the emotions I felt then. While I remember the pain and sadness of it all, I also remember the joy that this arduous process produced. I carried the twins for thirty-nine weeks! At birth, one weighed six pounds fourteen ounces and the other eight pounds seven ounces: two healthy babies. I, on the other hand, had to overcome acute renal failure, went home with a walker, and was assigned an in-home nurse. Eventually, I healed up and other than being sleep deprived, things were great! Or so I thought. When the girls were five-months-old, my stomach gave out and I required a double umbilical hernia repair. Those wounds healed and I was doing well for a while and then, BOOM! Another whammy! We were faced with yet another trial.

Another Trial - Hello, Discoid Lupus!

My Story. Decide what you believe regarding diet modification as a form of treatment for lupus. In June 2011, my husband relocated to Korea (we are a military family) and our girls and I were required to wait several months before joining him. While we waited, we moved from New York to Virginia and lived with my parents for several months. For one of those months, during the summer of 2011, my parents, my five-month-old twins, and I traveled to Germany to visit my brother.

If you are familiar with natural black hair and what it takes to maintain it, you may know that a very simple style to maintain and care for is braids. Especially when you're on vacation! It's all about low to no maintenance and that's exactly what I was looking for as a new mother of twins! So, off to Germany we went with my hair in nice, neat, low-maintenance braids! Natural black hair requires a lot of moisture especially when wearing a protective style such as braids. If the hair and scalp are not properly moisturized you can end up with a very dry and itchy scalp. Shortly after arriving in Germany, I noticed an itchy spot on my scalp. First thought? Put some braid spray on there and call it good! Unfortunately, the spray didn't help and the itching continued. After several days, it scabbed over and all I could think was, *this is not the sort of itching I'm accustomed to.*

By the end of summer, I had a small patch of scalp that was no longer growing hair. I decided I wouldn't stress about it. I had more pressing issues that required my attention, like a diagnosis of a double umbilical hernia that needed repair. So, I figured it would be best to address my itchy scalp once the girls and I joined my husband in Korea.

November 2011. The girls and I arrived in Korea and the itching became more intense. I remember telling my husband that my head felt as though I had bugs crawling under my scalp. It itched so badly it felt like my skin was crawling! My husband suggested that I not tell the doctor that part about the bugs, but that was the only way I could think to describe it. By this time, I had more than one bald patch on my head and they were spreading. As you can probably imagine, I was beyond freaked out.

Once I was processed into the medical care system in Korea, I was able to make an appointment with a dermatologist. As I waited for that initial appointment, I started conducting my own research consisting of endless Google searches in order to self-diagnose. Probably not the best idea, but I did it anyway. I found everything from alopecia to a YouTube video of a man pulling worms from his wife's scalp after their trip to some jungle in South America.

By March 2012, I'd seen the dermatologist at least twice and had a scalp biopsy that came back positive for discoid lupus. *Discoid what?!*

What Is Discoid Lupus?

Discoid Lupus Erythematosus (DLE) is an autoimmune disease and the most common form of lupus. It is associated with inflammation and scarring. Unlike systemic lupus erythematosus (SLE), that can affect any part of the body, DLE primarily affects the skin. Based on my research and personal experience, DLE "attacks" its victims from the neck up. People who have discoid lupus often develop sores or lesions on the face, scalp, and even in the ears. It is visible and often times disfiguring, leaving its "victims" feeling insecure and wounding their self-esteems.

According to the Lupus Foundation of America, an estimated 1.5 million Americans and at least five million people worldwide have a form of lupus. **The majority of Americans are not sure what kinds of treatments are generally prescribed to treat lupus.**

Here are some interesting statistics I discovered as I researched what Americans believe, or do not believe, about lupus:

- Roughly 6 in 10 individuals (58%) do not know how lupus is treated.
- About one-fifth (22%) say corticosteroids - Prednisone, 1 in 10 or fewer individuals say antimalarials - Plaquenil (9%), chemotherapy medications (8%), organ rejection drugs (7%), or something else (11%) are used to treat lupus.

This particular survey did not offer "food" or "dietary modification" as answer choices for possible treatments. Because this was a multiple choice question, it is possible that respondents who selected answer option 4, "Something Else," included those who believe dietary modifications to be a form of treatment.

Another striking take-away from the survey is that most Americans **do not** believe that lupus can be prevented. In fact, more than half (56%) overall did not agree with the statement that lupus can be prevented, while only 18% say the statement is true. [2]

Let's unpack all of this a little bit. So we've discussed what discoid lupus is and have referred to systemic lupus and how it differs from the discoid variant, but what is exactly is an autoimmune disorder?

When you hear the word autoimmune, two things should immediately come to mind. First, think about a person's body attacking itself and second, inflammation. Simply put, autoimmune disorders are when person's body begins to attack itself. Put another way, a person's body tissues are attacked by their own immune system. Essentially, they are abnormal immune responses to a normal body part. You see, our immune systems are indented to find and destroy foreign invaders in the body. People with autoimmune disorders typically have objects circulating in their blood that don't belong. These objects are identified as foreign invaders and the invasion causes inflammation.

How Do The Foreign Invaders Get Into The Bloodstream?

Sugar, wheat (gluten), barley, and rye, all have the ability to damage our intestinal lining. Our intestinal lining is not supposed to allow anything to pass through it into our blood streams. However, if the lining is damaged (also known as leaky gut), all sorts of goodies that shouldn't be out and about leak directly into the bloodstream.

Imagine your gut lining is like a tightly woven fence or a steel pipe carrying sewage. Let's go with the pipe full of sewage analogy. When damaged (some people's linings are more easily damaged than others), it's as if the pipe rusted through creating a hole for the sewage to leak into the clean water (the bloodstream) and the result is the development of an autoimmune disorder! It's really as simple as that!

When toxins make their way into the bloodstream an autoimmune reaction is triggered. Our antibodies, like soldiers, march out to attack the foreign invaders and sometimes they get confused! It is their confusion that causes us pain and illness. Of course, the antibodies mean well, but in their confusion, they attack the "bad guys" (the toxins) AND unfortunately the "good guys" (the parts of our bodies that didn't do anything wrong to deserve the war being waged against them) too.

What Causes Autoimmune Disorders To Manifest Themselves?

Hereditary: Some individuals are predisposed to autoimmune disorders because it's in their genes. Heredity is a factor, even if the trait skips a generation or two.

Permeable gut lining: As described earlier, a damaged gut lining allows particles mistaken for foreign invaders to leak into the bloodstream triggering an autoimmune flare. A physician once told me that it's best to avoid barley, wheat, and rye because those grains, based on the way they are processed today, are intestinal lining destroyers. Refined sugar is a gut lining destroyer too.

Drug-induced: According to *Toxicology*, an international journal known for its focus on the mechanisms of toxicity, drug-induced lupus (DIL) looks a lot like SLE clinically. The primary difference being that patients with DIL fully recover after the offending medication is discontinued. Incidentally, DIL has been reported as a side-effect of long-term therapy with over 40 medications. [3]

Medications prescribed: The dermatologist immediately prescribed me Clobetasol, a topical anti-inflammatory. As I recall, I applied it at least twice a day to the smooth spots on my scalp. During that first visit I received cortisone injections in my head to help reduce the inflammation. Between the Clobetasol and the cortisone injections, I got some relief from feeling as though my skin was crawling, until my biopsy results came back.

Once the biopsy came back positive for inflammation, I was prescribed Plaquenil, an oral antimalarial, also known as hydroxychloroquine. The side effects of Plaquenil are retinal toxicity and potential irreversible vision loss. So, before starting on this medication I had to see an ophthalmologist for a baseline retina exam. I was on the medication for just over a year and was required to go in for periodic retina checks to ensure there were no changes to my vision.

I knew I couldn't be on that antimalarial forever for a couple of reasons. First, I wasn't interested in playing around with potentially losing my eyesight! And second, we had two embryos left from our IVF experience and there was no way I could be on that medication and hope for a safe and healthy embryo transfer. In fact, my reproductive endocrinologist advised me to get healthy and eat organic whenever I could. I made it my mission to come off all of the medication.

A New Report

By August 2013, my family returned to the USA from Korea. It had been several months since I'd had any autoimmune attacks. After a visit to my new physician and some blood tests, I learned that my body had stopped attacking itself and there were no indications that I needed to remain on the Plaquenil. My dosages were decreased until I was completely off of it. Triumph! Mission complete!

How Did I Do It?

I adopted a plant-based diet and by doing so was able to "turn off" my autoimmune problem and stop medication all together! As I shared earlier, shortly after I was diagnosed with discoid lupus, I went on a quest in search of a natural solution to my problem. I am a true believer in the healing power of foods and was excited when I stumbled upon Jill Harrington's website and her book, *The Lupus Recovery Diet*. From her story of suffering and recovery from SLE, I learned that it is possible to ditch the medication and put an autoimmune disorder where it belongs—in the rearview mirror!

> "The food you eat can be either the safest and most powerful form of medicine or the slowest form of poison."
> ~ANN WIGMORE

The four things that I decided to remove from my diet immediately were salt, oil, sugar (SOS), and all animal protein including fish and eggs. It's true, by eating SOS free, I successfully put that annoying discoid lupus into remission. People often asked me how I could eat plant-based and wondered if I missed eating things that "taste good," as if plant-based eating can't taste good. My answer? It's easy! When you are in enough pain, you'll make the necessary lifestyle changes required to make the pain go away. In my case, I just preferred eating plant-based foods over potentially losing my eyesight from the antimalarial medication or walking around with bald itchy lesions on my head. To tell you the truth, I was more concerned with the latter.

When you are in enough pain, you'll make the necessary lifestyle changes required to make the pain go away.

These days, I'm not perfect when it comes to adhering to my autoimmune-friendly eating habits. I'll be the first to admit that. However, when I stray, I find I ask myself and those closest to me, "Why the heck am I'm eating like I'm invincible? Why am I not freaked out like I used to be when I was first diagnosed and learned how to fix the problem naturally with food?" These questions, and their answers, typically get me back on track.

My Thoughts On What Triggered My Discoid Lupus Symptoms

I can't say that it was hereditary simply because no one in my family, grandparents included, has a history of autoimmune disorders except for one of my younger sisters who developed a hyperactive thyroid in college. I truly believe what I like to call the "big three" happened to me: increased stress, lack of sleep, and lack of exercise.

After a C-Section, a double hernia repair, being up at all hours of the night caring for infant twins while my husband was away for four months, it's clear that the "big three" were my reality for a while. Even so, I am so thankful for my parents who were a tremendous help during those four months that I was a single-mom geographically. They helped me care for the girls. They waited on me when I laid in bed recovering from hernia repair surgery. They helped feed one baby, while I fed the other. Occasionally, they took one twin at night so that I could get some rest. Although they were always willing and able to help, I didn't want to ask them to help all of the time. As a result, I naturally found myself painfully exhausted and in terrible need of sleep.

Sometimes, I wonder if my symptoms were drug-induced as my IVF journey required a host of medications and hormones. Just something I've pondered.

How To Determine If You Have An Autoimmune Disorder
- Antinuclear antibody (ANA) test
- Autoantibody test
- Organ functions test
- Complete blood count (CBC)
- Comprehensive metabolic panel
- C-reactive protein (CRP)
- Erythrocyte sedimentation rate (ESR)
- Urinalysis
- Biopsy

The methods of autoimmune disorder detection I experienced were ANA tests, biopsy, and ESR. ESR is a non-specific blood test that helps detect the presence of inflammation in a person's body, but doesn't indicate exactly where the inflammation is or what's causing it. It is usually used in conjunction with other tests. While I don't recall the details of my ESR, I will never forget my biopsy experience! The dermatologist gave me a shot or two of a local anesthetic directly into my scalp before taking a hole puncher-like tool that was razor sharp and punched it into my scalp twice, removing the suspected inflamed tissue. Yeah, kind of hard to forget that.

The presence of elevated antinuclear antibody (ANA) levels in the blood is another indicator of an autoimmune disorder. ANAs are naturally present in the body, but only in small amounts. When ANA levels are above the normal range it suggests the presence of an autoimmune disorder.

What You Can Do To Transition To Autoimmune Friendly Eating Habits

Several of the points listed below are what I implemented in my healing, and are adapted from the book, *Eating for Energy* by Yuri Elkaim.

Take control of your thoughts. There is an old saying, *"What you think about, you bring about."* Shift your negative thoughts to thoughts of positivity and healing. This is not always easy when suffering from a painful ailment, but it is way better than contributing to the pain with negative thoughts.

Harden your immune system. You can achieve this by reducing your stress levels, increasing your hours of consecutive sleep, and exercising. Cortisol is the "stress hormone." When cortisol is released into our bloodstreams it weakens our immune systems, inhibits the actions of our white blood cells, increases the chances of infection, and even promotes weight gain. So, it's best to bust the stress hormone! How? Remove or manage your stressors, exercise, go for regular massages, or body work. Do whatever relaxes you.

Increase your intake of raw plant-foods. Begin by reducing the processed foods you keep in your pantry. If it's not there, you can't eat it. Increase the amount and variety of raw foods you keep on hand and consume them throughout the day.

Transition away from a meat-based diet. Meat is a tough one for some people to part with. In my personal experience, I quit cold turkey because eliminating meat was much less painful than my symptoms. My research revealed that cutting animal protein out of my diet would prevent my body from attacking itself. If you are unable to quit cold turkey, gradually eliminate meat in this order: red meat, pork, chicken, and fish. If you're worried about getting enough protein, just consider the gorilla. Gorillas are herbivores and look how strong they are!

Transition away from dairy. Consider this: humans are the only mammals that drink milk beyond infancy, AND it's milk from a different species to boot! Eliminating animal protein from the diet includes ditching the dairy. Who wants to keep eating foods that encourage mucus production and congestion anyway?!

When it comes to healing the body, I am a true believer in the power of food. Overcoming my discoid lupus symptoms with nutrition was not my first rodeo. In high school, I suffered from inexplicable disfiguring allergic reactions. My lips would swell so badly my parents supported my staying home from school to avoid the shame and embarrassment. To keep me from having to take an antihistamine every night, my mom took me to an iridologist who put me on a plant-based diet (minus hard boiled eggs) for a year and a half which resulted in total body healing for me.

In 2013 and 2014, I became lax with my tried and true lupus recovery diet; my symptoms returned. I needed to get back on the right track quickly. So, in early 2015, I committed to a medically supervised 9-day water-only fast at the TrueNorth Health Center in Santa Rosa, California. Under the care of Dr. Michael Klaper, I experienced total healing! My discoid lupus symptoms vanished and I returned home feeling amazing!

Now that you've heard my story, what do you believe regarding diet modification as a form of treatment for lupus? Better yet, what do you believe about the human body's ability to heal itself?

On the journey of life, there will be ups and downs, bumps and bruises. Some will be expected and others will come as shocks or surprises. Life is not always easy and we don't control everything that happens to us, but there are some things we can control. Without question, we are in control of our attitudes of mind and how we nourish our bodies. Our thoughts and our fuel play significant roles in keeping our bodies healthy. No matter how tough the road ahead may seem, you are capable of traveling it! Take one step at a time and allow your body to heal from the inside out! You've got this!

Suggested Reading or Audio-Book:
- Michael Pollan's *In Defense of Food: An Eater's Manifesto*
- *The Lupus Recovery Diet: A Natural Approach to Autoimmune Disease by* Jill Harrington
- *Eating for Energy: Transforming your life through living plant-based whole foods*
- Yuri Elkaim, BPHE, CK, RHN
- *Eat to Live* by Dr. Joel Fuhrman
- Borchers, A. T., Keen, C. L., & Gershwin, M. (2007). Drug-Induced Lupus. *Annals of the New York Academy of Sciences, 1108*(1), 166-182.

Supplements I Take to Reduce Stress and Inflammation:
CuraMed | Natural Calm

Other Resources:
TrueNorth Health Center for medically supervised water fasting
www.healthpromoting.com
Dr. Michael Blotner, Reproductive Endocrinologist | www.westchesterfertility.com
IVF Support Group | www.facebook.com/groups/917354475043161/
www.allisonmarschean.com/my-favorite-things.html
Ask your physician about an intestinal permeability sample collection kit to test the condition of your intestinal lining. Genova Diagnostics, www.GDX.net, is one option.

Music - *Artists and the songs that kept me focused and positive during my IVF journey*
Josh Wilson: Before the Morning, Laura Story: Blessings
Kutless: What Faith Can Do, NEEDTOBREATHE: Shine On

THANK YOU

I'd like to first thank my Lord and Savior, Jesus Christ, for giving me something to write about. A huge thank you to my husband, Vince, who fully supported me in this endeavor. You never once questioned my desire to make a go of this even though I've never officially published anything before. Thank you so much for encouraging me to take this opportunity! That means so much to me! To my daughters Brynn, Piper, and Jordan, may you always know that you are loved beyond measure and were meant to be. To my sister, Kirsten, and mom, Harriett, we are a triple braided cord! We will walk hand in hand across somebody's stage! To my West Point classmate, Jewell. Thank you for thinking of me when you learned about this project! Finally, to my parents, Dennis and Harriett, who taught me to do my best at everything I put my hand to!

~ Allison Marschean

ACUPUNCTURE TO MY RESCUE

PEOPLE HAVE CALLED ME A SURVIVOR,

I RESENT THAT LABEL, I PREFER LESSON-LEARNER.

WITH THIS PERSPECTIVE, I WAS ABLE TO OVERCOME

MANY ADVERSITIES AND WIN THE FIGHT

TOWARDS BETTER HEALTH AND WELLNESS.

by Jenna Knight

Registered Acupuncturist, R.Ac

Jenna Knight

Jenna was born and raised in East Vancouver, BC, Canada. Being born into a family rich in adversity meant that she learned to fight for her health and well-being from a very early age. She completed her undergraduate studies at Thompson Rivers University, where she acquired an associates' degree in a variety of studies that included, health sciences, nutrition, sociology, and psychology. Jenna also completed the three-year registered acupuncturist program at the International College of Traditional Chinese Medicine, in April 2017 and wrote her licensing exams with the CTCMA in the fall of 2017.

She further expanded her studies in April 2017 and completed a two-week internship in Taiwan, at the Taipei Tzu Chi Buddhist Hospital. She attended lectures on (YNSA) scalp acupuncture with Dr. Sunfish Lee, the theory of acupuncture with Dr. Hsu, Tui Na with Dr. Huang, and gynecology with Dr. Chen (head of the TCM department). In the student clinic, Jenna thrived when treating the elderly, youth at risk, or individuals with emotional imbalances. Jenna has an interest in maintaining a hands on approach, so she advanced her training in the Chinese style massage called Tui Na and completed a five day (60 hour) intensive course in Vancouver, in September 2017.

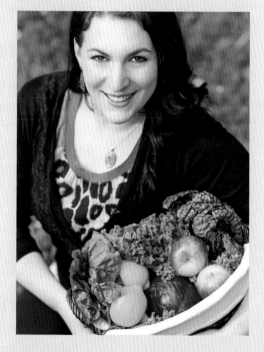

By October 2017, Jenna became a published wellness writer with her first article being published, in *Medicinal Roots Magazine* on insomnia. In her spare time Jenna enjoys being in the mountains, where she explores all of the beautiful hiking trails in BC. Here, she can take advantage her passion for photography, while also experiencing nature. Jenna also enjoys her motorcycle and spends time riding on sunny days.

WWW.ZENFLOWERACU.COM
fb: JennaKAcupunctureJourney
li: jenna-knight-70585baa
t: jknightacu

I am sixteen-years-old, and I'm sitting at the coffee table eating my dinner in a plume of cigarette smoke, which has stained our white walls to an orange tinged hazy color. I look down at my meal; there are no vegetables present on my plate, only different tones of beige, and textured mush. We eat a lot of meat and potatoes: it's hard to find a fresh vegetable in our home other than iceberg lettuce. Our food is tasteless, boring, and bland. Other than salt, we don't have anything to season our food with, not even pepper. It's hard to eat because I feel so congested, fighting off yet another cold. I'm sick all the time and it seems like I can never get better. It was pneumonia last month, bronchitis before that, and pleurisy before that. Now I have a gray stain coming through my throat to the skin on my neck, from inhaling so much second hand smoke in a small closed room. I don't have a bedroom or a bed; I sleep on the floor in the living room, so it's practically impossible to escape the smoke.

Dinner is done, dishes are done, my homework is done, and now it's time for bed. I lay down on the floor to go to sleep. Tonight I'm going to bed with yet another stomach ache. I haven't had a bowel movement in five days, but I am used to the pain as this is a regular problem for me. My dad solves my digestive problems with a bag of prunes from the bulk foods department of the local Superstore. *Crash! Smash*! I wake up to the sound of the door being broken off of its hinges. It's 3:00 a.m. and my older brother is having a bad trip while he is coming down from snorting way too much cocaine. He's stumbling all over the place, pupils wide and wild, as blood gushes from his nostrils and splashes across my face. My brother is crying, twitching uncontrollably, and asks for a hug. I give his massive bodybuilder physique a hug and embrace a hot yet cold body soaked in sweat, which leaves me clammy. He's asking my dad to help him dial the phone number for the drug dealer to get him more cocaine. His drug fix arrives, and and just like that, this nightmare is over, for tonight at least, anyway.

Morning comes, and I feel like death, as I try to get ready for school. My dad feeds me oil soaked eggs, hash browns, and bacon, with enough grease to stop my heart right there. The exhaustion from being woken up in the night and coping with the rush of adrenaline caused by fear and emotional distress has left me feeling like I'm running on an empty battery. The drive to school is quiet and cold, I'm sure my dad is exhausted too. This routine is normal for him, as he also has drug problems, but he thinks I'm not aware of his habits. However, I have become too aware and I know it, constantly using my imaginary antennas to sense what terrible events are going to happen to me before they occur. I know this is not normal; I know you shouldn't suffer so much at the hands of your loved ones, but I'm only a teenager, my voice is drowned out by the chaos of our daily life and my cry for help often goes unheard.

After school is done for the day, I go to work at the local pet store in their animal department until 9:30 p.m. I have yet another urinary tract infection but I refuse to let it affect my job, so I push through the discomfort and pretend I'm okay. I have had a urinary tract infection every month for years now, making me heavily reliant on a truck load of antibiotics to control the burning, urgency, bloody urine, and pain. All things being considered, my after school job is great. It is almost my safe haven and a much needed escape from my tumultuous home life, plus, I love animals. I discover my purpose very quickly through this first job; I am my best self when I am helping people. It is here that I meet a nice boy and we start dating, he is much older than me, and that makes people nervous. He is teaching me what I already magically knew in my heart, he is showing me with every action what love is supposed to be. When my dad picks me up from work, he immediately lets me know that he is not happy about my boyfriend. He explains to me that I am his "property" until I'm twenty-one-years-old and that all my boyfriend wants from me is to fuck me and then get rid of me, then adding another remark that this is all that any man will ever want from me. My inner voice snaps back immediately with a *how dare you talk to your daughter like that,* but no sound comes out of my mouth because it would be wasted breath. I can tell that my dad is trying to stomp out my light, everything that is positive about me, he is trying to control with some form of abuse. I know that if I stay in this toxic environment, I will never grow. I'm taking abuse from every angle. I feel like a fish in a shallow bowl of water; where each day some twisted kid walks by to drip a drop of bleach into my water. Eventually, I'm swimming in toxic water, with no escape, doomed to wither away.

I decide to escape from home. I wait until my dad goes out, then I leave by jumping out of a window with just a backpack. I know I'll be okay and I know that no one will look for me, as I have left a threatening note that I will expose my dad to the police if he even dares to search for me. My dad knows that I will stay true to my word, so I know I'm now safe from his grasp. Even though I know I am free, I still have many wounds to heal. My boyfriend sees that my emotional wounds still bleed because even the simple things are sometimes hard: a trip to the doctor's office results in terror and panic. I know it's normal to fear healing, healing requires change, and change can be scary for even the best of us. I'm used to the feeling of being scared though, so I've decided that instead of transforming slowly like a caterpillar becoming a butterfly, I'm going to rise from hot embers and ash like a phoenix and take control of my life.

In the first year away from home, I committed to seeing a counsellor on a regular basis, in an attempt to close my emotional wounds. After that, I spent each year working on one aspect of myself. It wasn't easy, but I always had my one person there to hold my hand and encourage each step that I took. I found a naturopath and began to address my digestive troubles, which were easily fixed with proper nutrition and minor adjustments. With the help of my naturopath, we were able to isolate foods that I was sensitive to and eliminated each one from my diet. This meant no gluten, dairy, or sugar. I had to be very aggressive with my Western medicine doctor and really push for a proper diagnostic work up for my intestinal troubles. I was told multiple times by doctors that I was normal and then labelled with "Nothing is wrong, it's all in her head." Finally after going through four family doctors, a urologist, and a gastroenterologist, I was given a diagnosis. During this time I experienced more blood draws than I can count, x-rays, ultrasounds, fluoroscopies, two urethroscopies with dilation, and a barium enema.

With this diagnosis I quickly learned that I had a type of intestinal disease called "Hirschsprung's Disease" and from the point of view held by my gastroenterologist, I would just have to live with the uncomfortable symptoms related to the disease. Now I was labelled with chronic illness and when Western medicine couldn't help me, I sought healing from traditional Chinese medicine to manage my symptoms. I consulted quite a few doctors about my digestive problems, and each one repeatedly told me that I would just have to accept living with the numerous uncomfortable symptoms that were associated with my intestinal disease. This was an unacceptable answer for me. I wouldn't allow a doctor to so easily label me with chronic illness and then simply dismiss me. So I pushed forward with the intention of bringing more "wellness" to my life. Through acupuncture, I was able to manage my intestinal disease and restore balance to my mind, body, and spirit. My naturopath suggested natural supplements to heal my intestinal lining, which ultimately boosted my immune system, and I never experienced a urinary tract infection again. In fact, after experiencing two urethroscopies with dilation, my urologist finally admitted that those procedures were unnecessary, as there was no physiological problem with the anatomy in my urinary tract. The last thing this urologist said before I left his office for the final time was not to worry, that all of my urinary problems would disappear after I get pregnant. If looks could kill, then hot magma would have erupted from my eye sockets and killed him on contact.

Each time I visited an allopathic doctor, I left their office feeling completely exhausted, and at times, it was hard to persist on my road to wellness. In contrast however, each time I visited my acupuncturist, naturopath, and counsellor, I left their office feeling more enlightened on ways that I could enhance my well-being. Suddenly, I looked around and realized that I had found myself a strong network of female healers who gave the gift of holistic wellness to their patients on a daily basis. My acupuncturist saw my interest in helping others and gradually coaxed me to consider a career in a holistic healing field. After speaking with her one day, it was as though a light bulb had suddenly turned on—I realized that I wanted to give this gift of wellness to those around me as well. She inspired me on a level that hit me in the heart, like a ray of sunshine hitting cold pavement. I already knew that I felt my best when I was helping others and I could not see anything more honorable in my mind than the act of helping people achieve good health. What seemed even more amazing to me was that these female healers would never get recognized for their countless efforts, but they provided an invaluable service to everyone they encountered within their community.

Now, fully inspired and completely fired up with a passion for helping people achieve a sense of well-being and healing, I have completed the licensed acupuncturist program and look forward to all that awaits me in the future. I have learned that acupuncture is like a key which unlocks doors that have disabled natural healing processes within our bodies. This key gives the human body the ability to heal itself. This effect may be hard to imagine, but note that it has been well documented, as acupuncture is one of the oldest forms of medicine on the planet, dating back 2500 years. [1]

An acupuncture treatment manipulates the flow of a life giving energy called "Qi" and the circulation of blood, which can restore health. Qi is accessed through the various acupuncture points along the meridians of the body by insertion with very fine needles. Research suggests by MRI results that acupuncture points have an acupuncture-brain-organ pathway and connection. [2,3] This means that needling specific acupuncture points has a therapeutic effect on targeted organs or organ systems.

Learning about acupuncture has helped me recognize the importance of preventing illness and has taught me to listen to my body for potentially serious signs of looming disease processes. The pain and discomfort that used to be normal for me is now a rarity. Just as I had recognized that my family home was toxic to my entire being, I was also able to see that living with discomfort was detrimental to my wellness. I knew that pain was slowly draining my life force and bringing my life potential down. I simply wasn't willing to accept that concept and I wasn't willing to limit myself with labels.

By seeking out acupuncture, I have found a treatment that naturally activates my nervous system, allowing my body to increase the release of its own natural pain-killing chemicals. These pain-killing chemicals are called endorphins, and are known to be 200 times stronger than morphine, with zero negative side effects. My digestive problems are now almost non-existent, as acupuncture has had a positive effect on the physiology of my gastrointestinal tract. This effect includes acid secretions and motility, which in my case are particularly important. Living with Hirschsprung's Disease means that I have to stay on top of my intestinal motility and continuously promote a healthy intestinal tract. The symptoms that I was told to tolerate in Western medicine were in fact totally manageable and unnecessary.

Now, I live each day with the perspective that we should love life, and if we don't, then the only answer is a dash of courage and serious directional changes. I would remind people from a similar background to remember that your inner voice is your compass, it can direct you to places that are full of darkness or bring you to the light. So please speak to your inner self softly and remember to always fight for your wellness. You have to be your own private warrior on your individual journey to wellness, no one can help you more than you can help yourself. You don't ever have to accept any labels placed on you by society. You can be more than you ever expected to be. Your outlook and perspective are everything. They are the key to you living and leading a life of well-being and good health. Guide yourself somewhere beautiful.

> ## You don't ever have to accept any labels placed on you by society.

THANK YOU

First, and foremost, I would like to thank Ky-Lee for putting together such an amazing book, with so many talented and educated ladies. Secondly, I want to thank my husband, who is my partner, my teammate, my biggest supporter, and the love of my life. I will look for you in our next lifetime. Thirdly, I would like to thank my daughter, who has continued to surprise me and has inspired me to be more than I ever knew I could be. And lastly, I would like to thank Clara Cohen, my friend, my TCM doctor and acupuncturist, who gave me the push I needed to jump into a career that I absolutely love.

~ Jenna Knight

GREEN FUEL ON HER PLATE

Featuring

Sindy Ng

Samantha Cifelli

Margie Cook

The Plantiful Chef

HEALING FROM WITHIN

THE MOST IMPORTANT RELATIONSHIP TO NURTURE
IS THE ONE YOU HAVE WITH YOURSELF.

by Sindy Ng

BASc Nutrition and Food

Sindy Ng

Sindy is a nutritionist with a Bachelor of Applied Science in nutrition and food. She is currently studying holistic nutrition to become a certified nutritional practitioner, with plans to specialize in holistic health and women's wellness.

Sindy's passion for health and wellness emerged through her recovery from an eating disorder. After struggling for years to find love and peace with herself throughout high school and university, she has come to embrace a holistic lifestyle from all aspects, including whole food nutrition, fitness, and toxin-free products. Sindy is a huge advocate for addressing the root causes of health issues, not merely the symptoms. She values the relationships that physical, emotional, and mental health contribute to overall well-being. As a budding entrepreneur, her goal is to thrive in the natural health field, guiding people of all backgrounds to achieve ultimate health on a personal level.

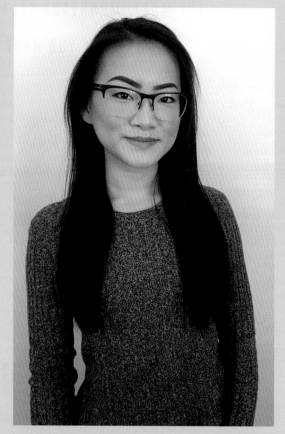

Sindy expresses her creativity through recipe development, food photography, and writing. She shares wholesome recipes and writes about informative health topics to inspire her readers to live an abundant lifestyle. Sindy has many aspirations, including creating recipe books, leading cooking and nutrition workshops, and counseling clients one-on-one. In the meantime, you can try some of her breakfast recipes in this chapter and follow along on her adventures through her blog and on Instagram.

WWW.HOLISTICFLOURISH.COM | SINDY@ HOLISTICFLOURISH.COM
ig: holisticflourish | fb: holisticflourish

My Past Shaped Me To Become A Stronger Version Of Myself

If someone told me five years ago that at age twenty-two I'd be writing a chapter in a book on women's health and wellness, I'd laugh. Although I love to cook and bake now, there was a time I wouldn't let myself taste certain foods, let alone make them for enjoyment. In fact, I struggled with an eating disorder for seven years— even throughout most of my university degree studying nutrition. Ironic, right? For me, food was incredibly stressful. The mere action of eating (what we all must do to survive) was horrifying. I didn't like eating foods if I didn't know the caloric content. I religiously tracked my meals and planned what I'd eat each day. I saw food as numbers. You could ask me how many calories were in a cup of carrots or a cup of grapes and I'd know.

"Let food be thy medicine, and medicine be thy food."

~ HIPPOCRATES

I reached out to my English teacher in the eleventh grade. She was the first person I ever talked to about my problem. I wasn't sure why, but I knew I needed to tell someone before I hurt myself with my binging and purging habits. I met with my school guidance counsellor, who set me up with a social worker. I talked with her for a few months before she had my doctor refer me to a hospital's eating disorder treatment program for adolescents. I spent part of the twelfth grade in the hospital's inpatient program with five other girls and completed my coursework with a teacher there. We had group activities, weigh-ins, check-ups, and weekend outings. I loved the girls, and we keep in touch to this day.

Once I turned eighteen-years-old though, I could make my own decision, and chose to leave the treatment program. I thought I was going to keep gaining weight, and hated that I was getting "fat." I had some tolerable days, bad days, and painful days. There were many points where I was so fed up with how my life was going, and I felt like I had no control. Eating disorders are a funny thing. You feel like you have some form of control when you reach your goal weight or your goal calories for the day. The truth is, you're the one being controlled. I was controlled by my mind for seven years. It was a tough cycle to break. Despite the support I had from friends or family members, I knew I had to be the one who *wanted* myself to recover. I needed to let go of everything I was afraid of. I needed to save myself so that I didn't have to suffer for the rest of my life.

Shortly after leaving treatment, I decided to study nutrition to become a registered dietitian and help other girls regain their health. I was battling my own challenges, but this was my motivation to achieve better health. I've always been the type of person who wanted to help others, even when I was the one who needed support. This was the time I had to select the programs and universities I wanted to attend in the fall. It was a precarious decision. I wasn't passionate about health and I had no interest in nutrition. What was I thinking? I didn't know, but I went along with my intuition.

Healing Myself First To Help Others

My road to recovery started when I discovered the benefits of a plant-based lifestyle on YouTube. I watched videos from a woman sharing how she healed from her eating disorder and became an athlete. I thought, *well, if she can eat all that food and look amazing, maybe I can too.* I transitioned slowly to a vegetarian diet and eventually adopted a plant-based lifestyle. It started with food, but I also became more conscious of the products I was using on my body and sought out brands that used natural ingredients. I quickly developed an interest in expanding my knowledge, and would constantly listen to podcasts on nutrition, health, and spiritual well-being, while reading books on these topics.

I started educating myself beyond what I learned in the classroom through literature, online resources, and documentaries. I volunteered for local and international non-profit organizations to apply my knowledge in sharing the benefits of a plant-based lifestyle. Currently, I'm working as a nutritionist at a health food store in Toronto, while studying holistic nutrition. As I learned more about natural health and complementary medicine, I realized that this field was more aligned with my values. Food should not only help us heal from disease, but help prevent or reduce the risks of developing them to begin with. We are what we eat, but we are also what we think and believe.

Healthy Intentions Create Healthy Food And Lifestyle Choices

Eating healthy doesn't have to be expensive, time-consuming, or boring. In fact, the breakfast recipes included in this chapter can be prepared quickly, stored, and used for several days, and can easily be adapted to suit your preferences. Breakfast is usually the first meal of the day, and many of us tend to rush in the morning and may skip breakfast, or pick up something on the way to work. I like to be prepared and make my day effortless by keeping my staples in the pantry and having foods assembled beforehand. Set aside some time for yourself in the morning to kick off the day with a positive intention. You'll find some tips in the recipes for make-ahead options and other tricks on saving time and money to ensure your day begins stress-free. The foods we choose affect not only how we physically look and feel, but also our mood, energy, and our choices for the rest of the day.

> Healthy doesn't mean perfect. To me, it means feeling happy, strong, and at peace with myself.

Consuming more whole, unprocessed foods allow me to feel more connected to what I put in my body. My goal is to inspire you to flourish through a holistic lifestyle that embraces mindful practices. Healthy doesn't mean perfect. To me, it means feeling happy, strong, and at peace with myself. To feel our best, we must nourish the mind, body, and spirit. Nutrition is merely one aspect of a healthy regime. Mental health, rest, movement, and social relationships all affect our state of well-being, yet they don't operate alone. Each of us only has one body to live in. Our bodies are our homes, so nurture them well.

THANK YOU

Mom and Dad, thank you for always being there for Tiffany, Norman, and I. Thank you for holding up through those painful years of me battling my eating disorder. I know how devastating it must've been for you, but I'm also glad that you've been so encouraging. Mom, you're always making comments about what I eat because you want me to be healthy, even though I remind you that I'm well educated on the topic. I know you do so because you love me. I hope to continuously make you proud. I'm aware the field of nutrition is quite vague to you, and you're occasionally concerned about how I could ever be successful in this field. I promise you that you have nothing to worry about.

Kevin, my partner and best friend, I can't thank you enough for being in my life. It wasn't long before we met that I became comfortable with myself for the first time since I could remember. I used to not leave the house or go to school without a full face of makeup on to cover my insecurities. I don't know how you did it, but you helped me learn to accept my "flaws" and be content with who I am and what I look like no matter what. I've never been happier. You've become a big part of my health journey and have supported me from the beginning. I'm thankful you're my go-to person who makes me laugh and feel incredibly lucky.

Ky-Lee, I'm so grateful to have met a strong, encouraging friend like you. I've looked up to you and admired all that you've achieved in the short time that I've known you. Thank you for giving me this opportunity to express myself and share a piece of my story to the world. I hope to lift and inspire as many women as you have.

~Sindy Ng

Breakfast

By Sindy Ng

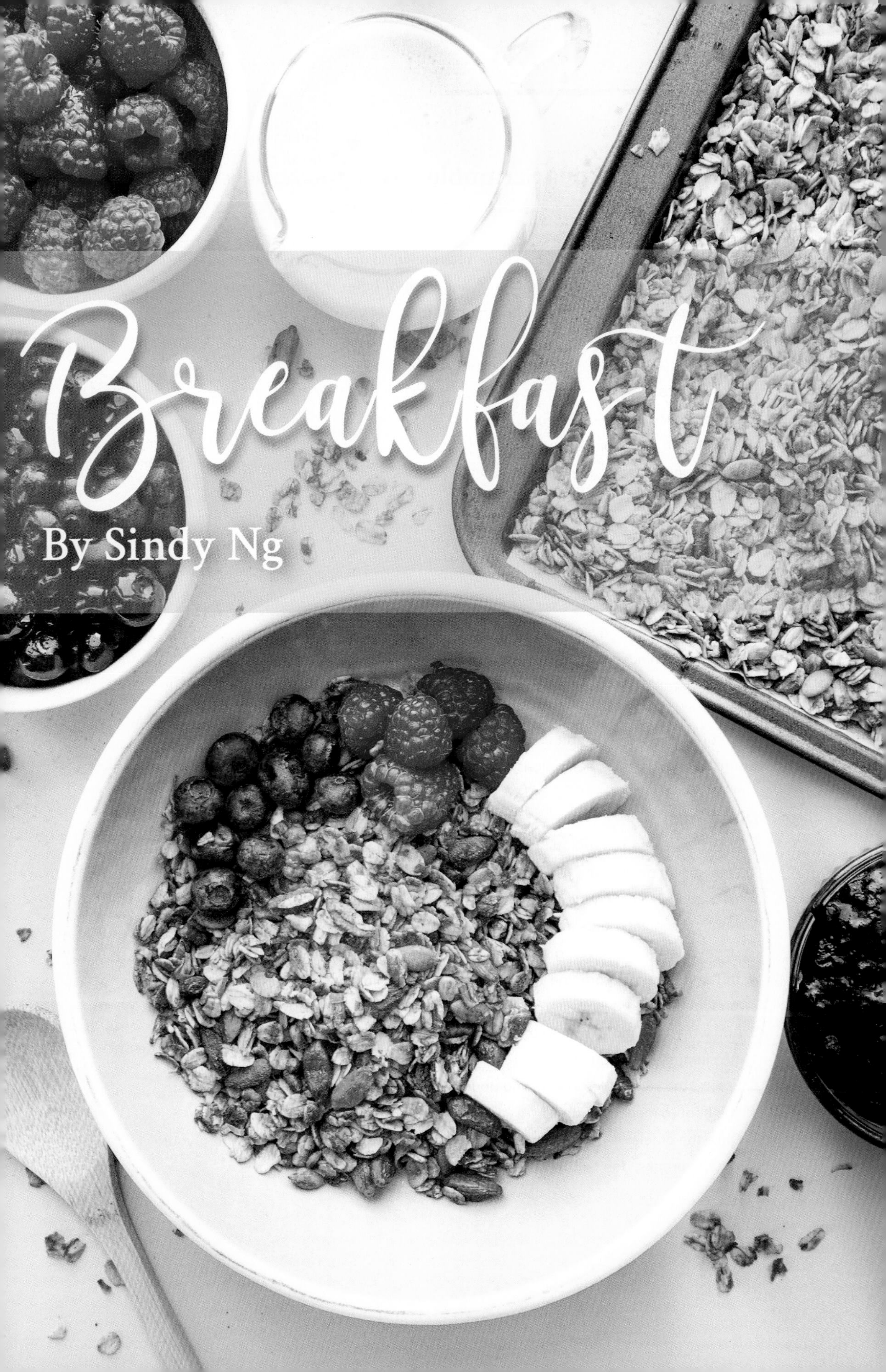

Savoury Chickpea Scramble

PREP TIME **10 minutes**
COOK TIME **15 minutes**
TOTAL TIME **25 minutes**

This chickpea scramble is a healthier alternative to traditional scrambled eggs. Loaded with protein, fiber, iron, folate, and several other minerals, chickpea flour is the base of this recipe. Enjoy with any vegetables of your choice. Add this to your next breakfast or brunch!

Ingredients

½ cup chickpea flour
½ cup filtered water or almond milk
¼ teaspoon turmeric
¼ teaspoon cumin
¼ teaspoon black pepper
¼ teaspoon paprika
½ teaspoon baking powder
2 tablespoons nutritional yeast
2 garlic cloves, minced
½ cup onion, minced
½ cup vegetables of choice, diced (red pepper, mushrooms, and baby spinach work well)
Pinch of pink Himalayan salt (optional)
Garnish: fresh herbs, green onions, avocado, or salsa (optional)

Directions

1. Dice the vegetables and mince the garlic and onion. Set aside.
2. Place a pan on medium heat. Add a pinch of salt and a teaspoon of coconut oil or avocado oil—just enough to sauté the vegetables.
3. Sauté the onions and garlic in the pan for 2 minutes before adding the other vegetables. If you're using spinach, add it at the end.
4. In the meantime, combine the chickpea flour, baking powder, nutritional yeast, and spices in a bowl.
5. Add water or almond milk to the dry mixture and combine well, ensuring there are no clumps of chickpea flour.
6. Spread the vegetables evenly and pour the batter over them to coat the pan. Turn the heat to medium-high.
7. Once the omelet is cooked through and the top is bubbling, you can flip it. If your omelet breaks, don't worry! Scramble it up.

8. Cook for another 10 minutes, mixing frequently. The chickpea batter should be cooked thoroughly.

9. Remove from heat and serve with green onions, avocado, salsa, or fresh herbs. Feel free to use it to top your toast!

Tips for an easy morning

Make a large batch of the dry ingredients, storing them in a glass jar in the pantry. When you want to make chickpea scramble, simply prepare your vegetables and then add equal amounts of water or almond milk to the dry mixture in a bowl. Change up the vegetables for variety.

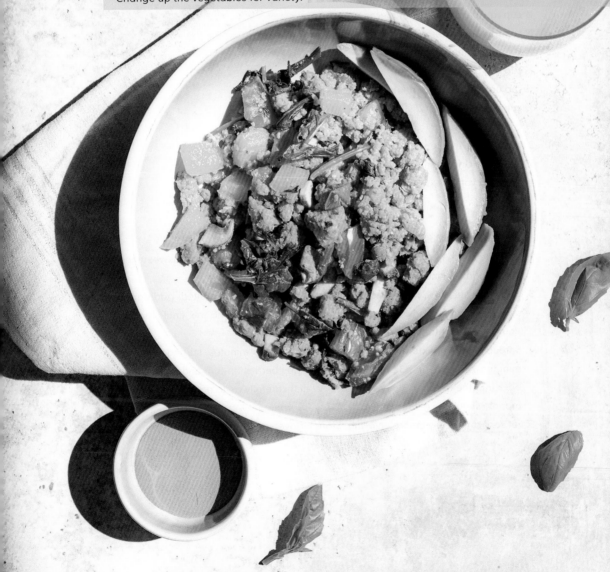

Super Seed Coconut Granola

PREP TIME **15 minutes**
COOK TIME **35 minutes**
TOTAL TIME **50 minutes**

Rich in omega-3 fatty acids, fiber, and antioxidants, this granola goes great with **Cashew Milk** (recipe on page 218) to make cereal. It also tastes delicious with yogurt and fruit. The recipe can easily be doubled and stored in your pantry for those mornings when you need some quick fuel!

Ingredients

2 cups rolled oats

½ cup raw pecan or walnut pieces

⅓ cup raw sunflower seeds

⅓ cup raw pumpkin seeds

⅓ cup goji berries

⅔ cup unsweetened coconut flakes (large flakes work best)

½ cup coconut oil

½ cup coconut sugar

2 tablespoons maple syrup or agave syrup

½ teaspoon cinnamon

1 teaspoon vanilla extract

Directions

1. Preheat oven to 350F.
2. Add rolled oats, pecans or walnuts, sunflower seeds, pumpkin seeds, unsweetened coconut flakes, and coconut sugar into a bowl. Mix to combine.
3. In a separate bowl, heat coconut oil in the microwave until melted. Add agave syrup, cinnamon, and vanilla extract into the coconut oil and mix until smooth. Pour the liquid into the dry mixture, stirring thoroughly.
4. Spread granola mixture onto a pan and bake for 35 minutes, stirring every 10 minutes. After the first 32 minutes, sprinkle goji berries on top, and put the pan back into the oven for 3 more minutes. Watch carefully as to not let it burn. The granola should be golden brown and very fragrant.
5. Let cool completely before enjoying. Store leftovers in a glass jar.

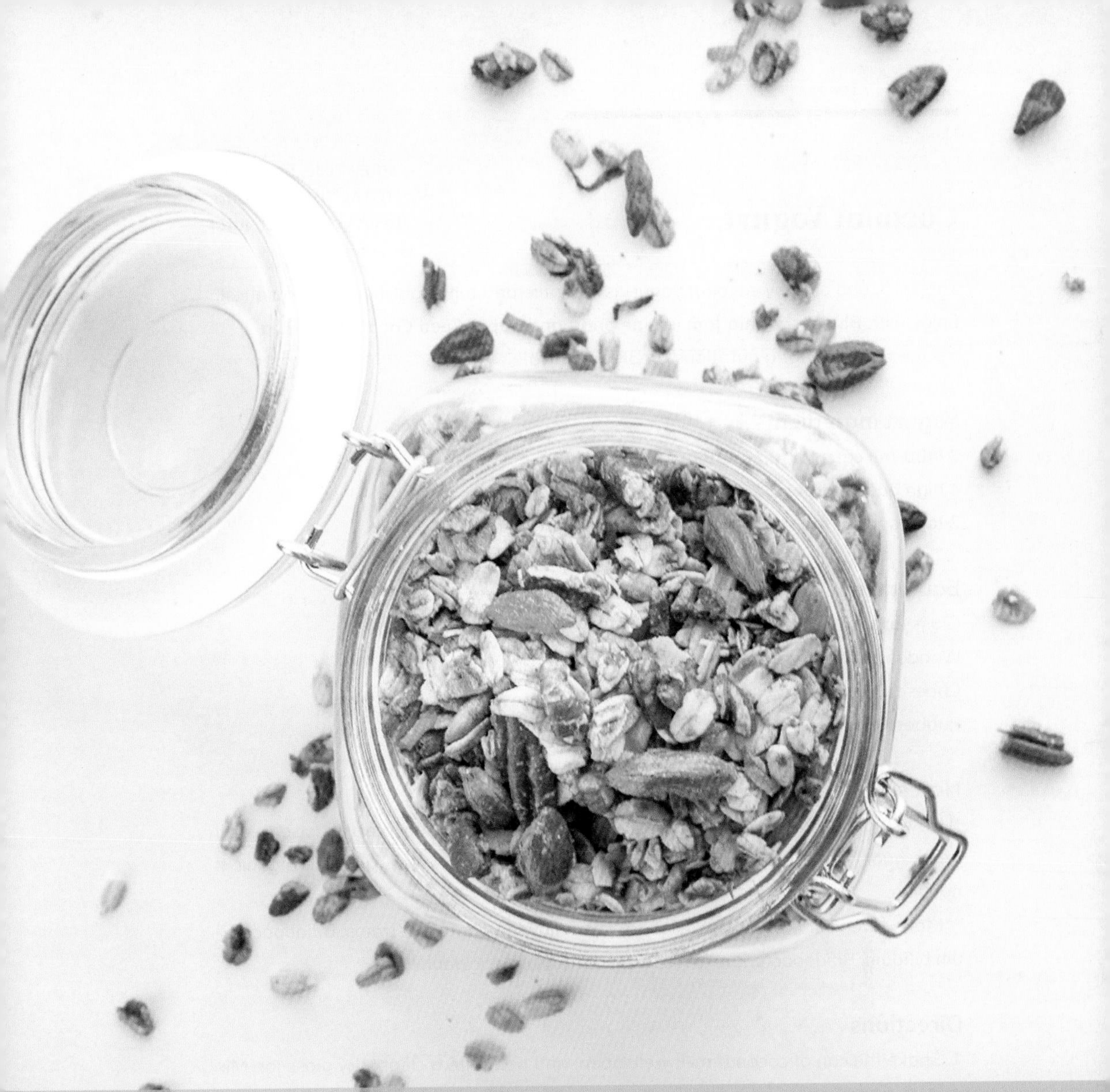
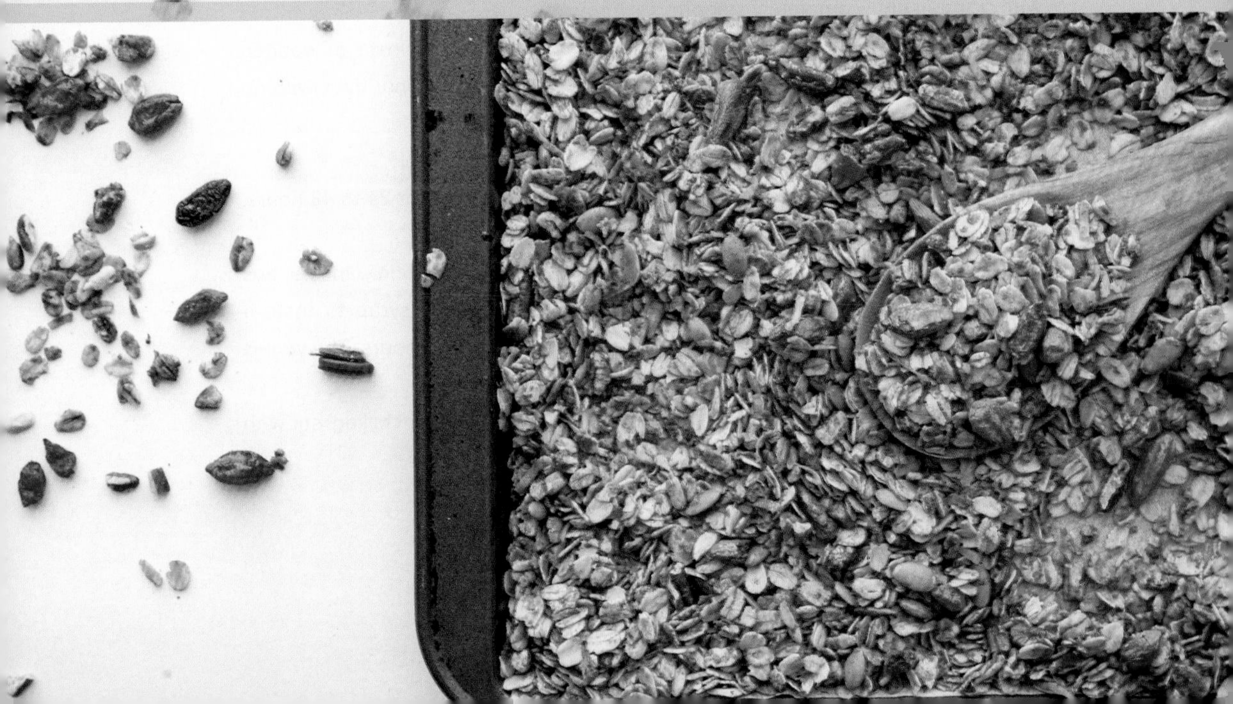

Coconut Yogurt

PREP TIME 5 minutes
TOTAL TIME 48 hours
(to let yogurt activate)

This thick and creamy coconut yogurt is versatile and full of gut-healthy probiotics! Enjoy with **Blueberry Chia Jam** (recipe prior) and **Super Seed Coconut Granola** (recipe to follow) for a nutritious breakfast parfait.

Yogurt ingredients

2 (400-ml) cans full-fat coconut milk*
4 high quality probiotic capsules**
2 tablespoons maple syrup

Equipment

Glass jar with lid
Wooden or plastic spoon
Cheesecloth
Rubber band

Notes

*Use full-fat coconut milk. The ingredient list shouldn't include water. It'll also work if it has guar gum added. Be sure it's not coconut milk "beverage." Choose organic if possible.

**Make sure your probiotic at least has the following bacterial strains: *Bifidobacterium bifidum, Bifidobacterium lactis*, and *Lactobacillus acidophilus*.

Directions

1. Shake the can of coconut milk well, open, and pour into a clean, dry glass jar. Mix with a spoon until completely smooth.
2. Carefully empty the probiotic capsules into the yogurt, using a plastic or wooden spoon. Stir until the probiotics are evenly distributed in the coconut milk, with no clumps. Add the maple syrup and mix well.
3. Cover the jar with a cheesecloth and secure with a rubber band.
4. Allow the yogurt to sit in a warm place away from direct light for 24 to 48 hours. The yogurt will be ready sooner in warmer climates.
5. After at least 24 hours, sample with a plastic or wooden spoon. Once it has reached your desired thickness and tanginess, stir in maple syrup to taste if desired. Secure the jar with a lid and refrigerate for at least six hours. The yogurt will thicken more.
6. Store yogurt in the fridge for up to two weeks. If it separates after chilling, stir with a spoon before enjoying.

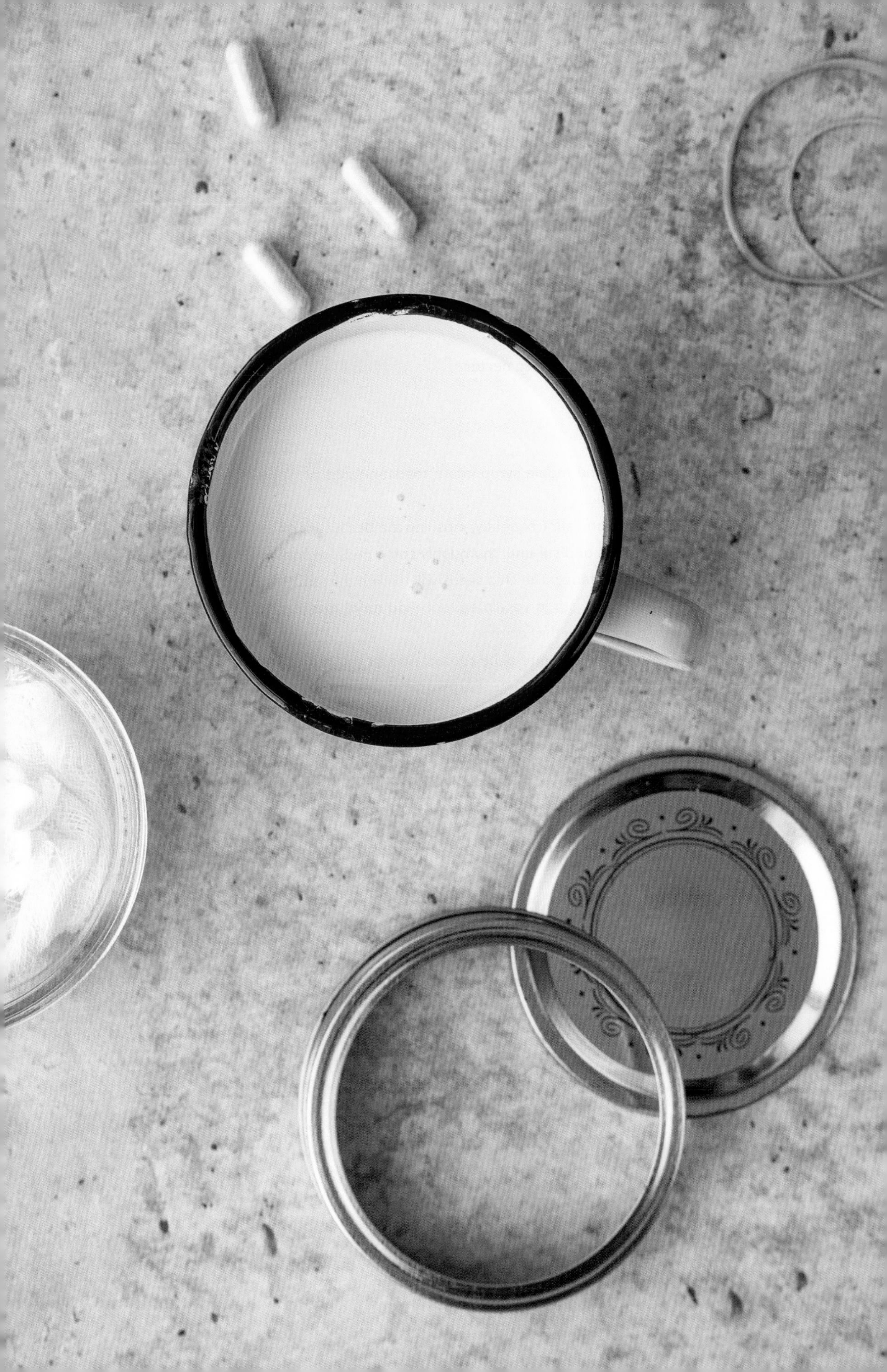

Blueberry Chia Jam

PREP TIME 2 minutes
COOK TIME 25 minutes
TOTAL TIME 27 minutes

Ingredients

3 cups fresh or frozen blueberries, strawberries, or raspberries

3 tablespoons pineapple juice or orange juice

3 tablespoons chia seeds, ground

1 tablespoon maple syrup or agave nectar

½ teaspoon vanilla extract

Directions

1. Place berries, juice, and maple syrup into a medium-sized pot on medium heat until it starts to bubble.

2. Reduce to a simmer and stir frequently, mashing the berries for about 5 minutes.

3. Add in the chia seeds and stir until thoroughly combined, for another 15 minutes to your desired consistency. The chia seeds will thicken the jam.

4. Remove from heat and stir in vanilla extract. Add more maple syrup if desired. Upon cooling, the jam will thicken more.

5. Transfer to an airtight container once cooled. Add to granola or yogurt. Store in the fridge for up to a week.

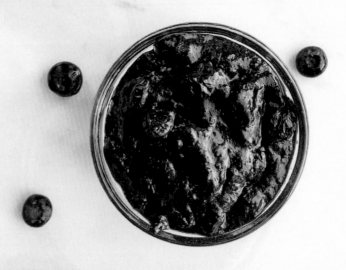

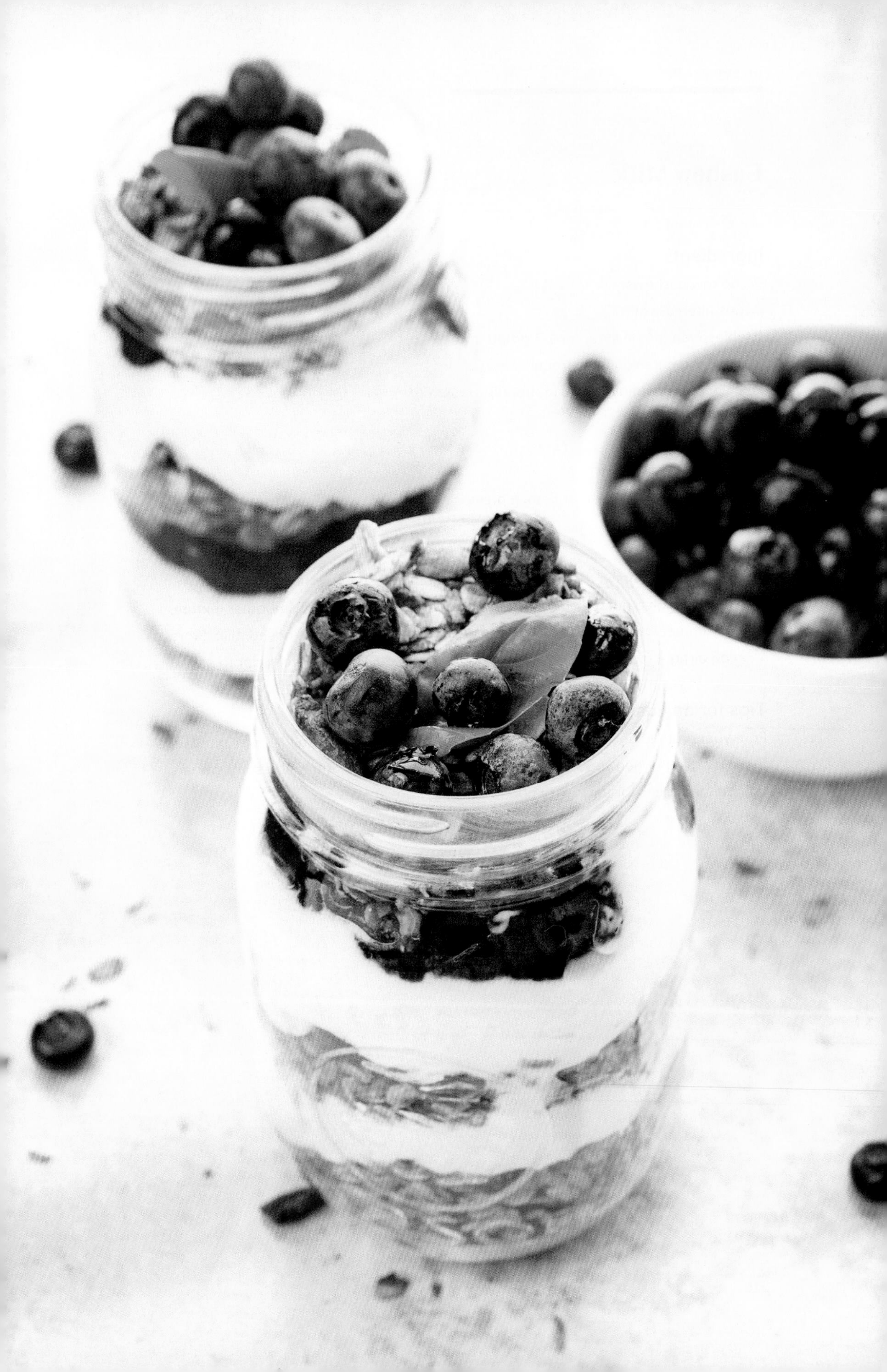

Cashew Milk

PREP TIME **2 minutes**
TOTAL TIME **5 minutes**

Ingredients

⅔ cup raw cashews

3 cups filtered water

1 tablespoon maple syrup or 1-2 pitted dates

½ teaspoon pure vanilla extract

Pinch of pink Himalayan salt (optional)

Equipment

Blender

Nut milk bag, coffee filter, or French press

Directions

1. Add all ingredients in the blender and blend on high speed until smooth.

2. Strain through a nut milk bag, coffee filter, or French press for a smoother texture.

3. Enjoy immediately in coffee, or in any recipes that call for plant-based milk. Store in an airtight glass jar. Keeps in the fridge for 4-5 days. Shake well prior to use.

Tips for an easy morning

Pour your granola and cashew milk into a bowl and eat it as cereal! It's so simple on those mornings when you have the granola already in your pantry. Add some berries and banana slices for that extra fiber and energy boost.

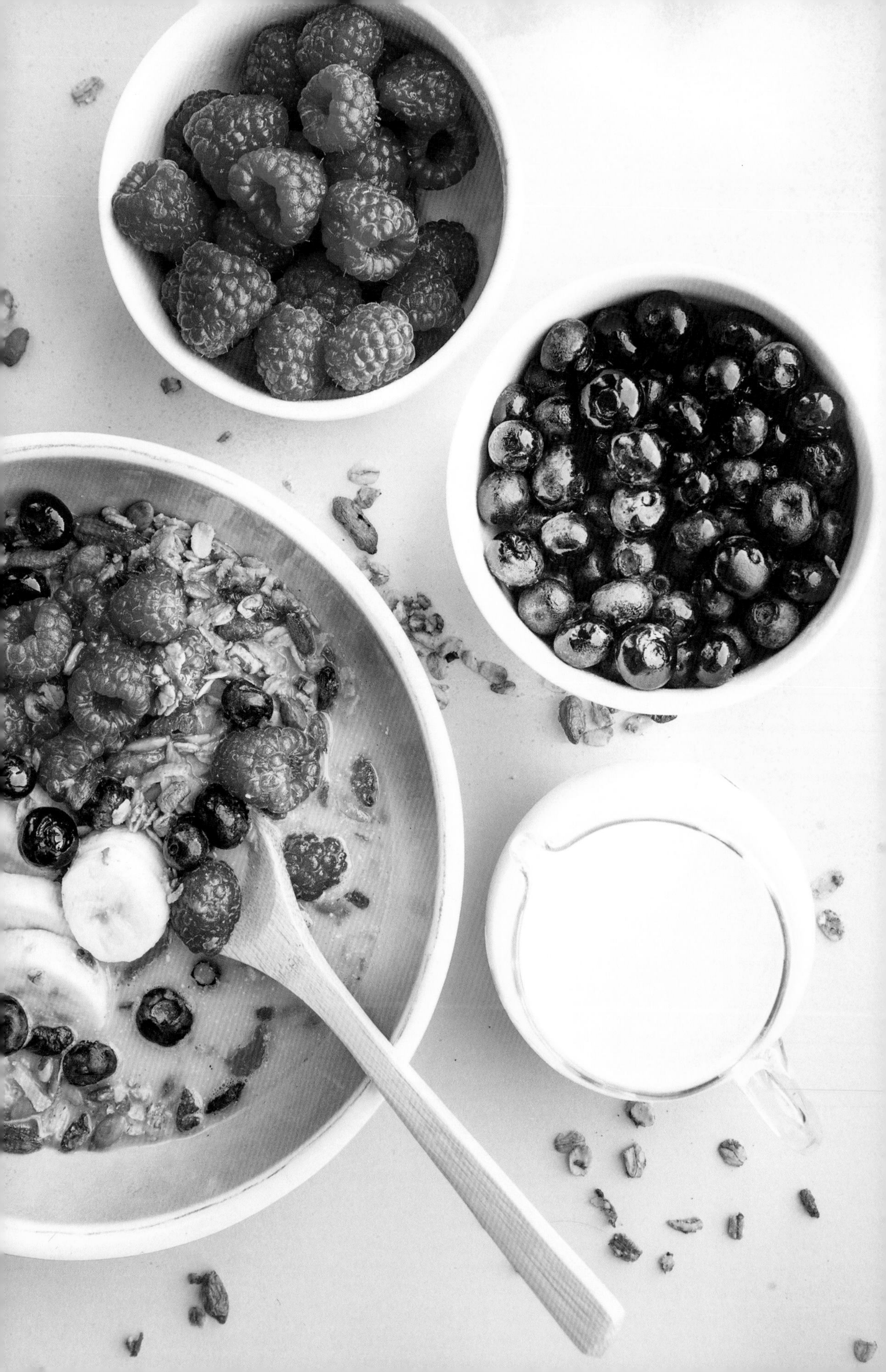

AN ITALIAN LESSON IN BALANCE

THE BEST FOOD IS COOKED WITH LOVE.

by Samantha Cifelli

MSc in Nutrition

Samantha Cifelli

Samantha is a nutritionist, professional writer, and certified life coach. She has her Bachelor of Science degree in nutrition and dietetics and a Master of Science in nutrition. Samantha has a passion for food, nutrition, and cooking and loves to help her clients achieve healthy living and a well-balanced, yet tasty, diet by utilizing her skillset in the kitchen with the knowledge of science and nutrition. She is known by her clients for her loving, sweet, and caring nature and her calm, attentive, and personalized approach. You can learn more about Samantha and her services by visiting her website at www.samanthacifelli.com, where she has an array of recipes, blogs, and links to her social media accounts.

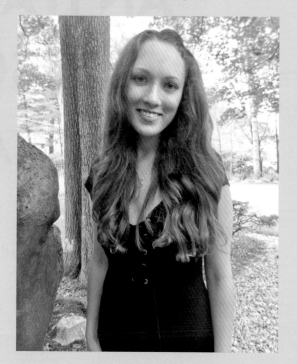

WWW.SAMANTHACIFELLI.COM
ig: samanthacifelli | fb: samanthacifelli-coach | t: samanthablaise2

Growing up in an Italian household in New Jersey, I was infused with a love of family, food, and cooking from an early age. Every meal was home cooked by my lovely mother; every holiday was a feast. Looking back, perhaps I took my norm as a young child for granted. My parents were still married at the time, and holidays were regularly celebrated at our house filled with family members from both sides of the family. If an outsider looking in were asked to describe my family, perhaps this individual would use such adjectives as "loud" or "crazy." If you were to ask me, however, I would simply say "love."

"Your first wealth is health."
~ Ralph Waldo Emerson

Italians are synonymous with food, and my family is and was no different. The culture is known for its delicious, homey cooking. Meals such as spaghetti and meatballs, chicken parmigiana, and penne alla vodka perhaps come to mind. While these and other Italian American dishes were no doubt a part of my upbringing, they were not the be all end all.

Growing up, I was regularly exposed to more Mediterranean diet style dishes. There were plenty of vegetable dishes, vegetable and bean salads, fruits for snacking or in place of desserts, fish, and whole grains in place of processed grains. The only drinks you would find in our fridge were water, low fat milk, and juices. There was no soda. In fact, I did not try my first soda until fifth grade. I did not enjoy it then, and I have yet to acquire a taste for it, something I thank my mother for, as she never introduced my brother or me to the beverage, nor created this sense of resistance towards it as some families do, by only offering sodas as treats or for "special occasions." Perhaps you can perceive a sense of balance in my upbringing. My mother never told me "no" at the grocery store to foods I wanted; yet, I still somehow was instilled with an overall healthy or well-rounded diet: less processed foods, more whole foods.

Whether you attribute it to genetics, my environment growing up, innate talent, or some combination of all three, I found myself a natural cook as a young child onwards. I remember making French toast for my friends after sleepovers. It was the best they ever had, they would tell me. I used to, and still do, dream of having my own cooking show and would put on shows in my kitchen. During car rides with my mother, I would fantasize recipe ideas, eagerly anticipating the next trip to the grocery store so I could purchase my ingredients and bring my recipes to life.

The aforementioned had all set the stage for my new found passion of nutrition, the science behind food. Though I only truly discovered my interest in science as a freshman in college, it makes sense as to why I felt called to this path. Food, in a sense, has always been my life. From family gatherings, to home cooked meals, to a natural instinct in the kitchen, to my mother's interest in health and purchasing organic foods for our family, and to, finally, a natural sense of balanced meals and whole foods that I have always been exposed to, the stage had been set for me to take this all a step further through my studies and working with clients: my mark of change in this vast universe.

My food mantra is this: Keep it simple, smart, and delicious. Food is an integral part of our existence. We owe it to ourselves to eat that which gives us pleasure and is enjoyable. Unfortunately, our taste buds seem to have been corrupted by processed sugars, chemicals, and unnatural growing processes. However, we can retrain our brains through the consumption of whole foods: fruits, vegetables, nuts, seeds, whole grains, herbs, spices, and healthy fats such as coconut oil and olive oil. By sticking to simple, whole, nutritionally-dense foods, we let go of our addictive qualities to processed foods and sugars as we nurture ourselves wholly: body, mind, and soul.

Authentic Italian cuisine is known for its taste; yet, it is the simplicity within its recipes, the quality of its ingredients, and the secret ingredient of love which bring forth an understated finesse to the final product. The lunch recipes of this chapter are all inspired by the makeup of authentic Italian and Mediterranean cuisine. They are also all time and budget friendly, as healthy, delicious foods do not require hours in the kitchen or a hefty supermarket bill. Lastly, there is a focus on the element of color and its relationship to health. The rays of color are not only pleasing to the eye, allowing us to eat with our eyes first, before food even reaches our taste buds, but each also provides various health benefits. It can be beneficial to aim for variety within the color spectrum as a means to eating a healthy, well-balanced diet.

Blue, purple, and deep red fruits and vegetables such as blackberries, blueberries, and eggplant are associated with the antioxidants called anthocyanins and pro-anthocyanins. These are optimal for heart and brain health. Cruciferous greens including green cabbage and broccoli contain isothiocyanates and indoles which are thought to prevent cancer by producing enzymes that clear toxins from the body. Leafy greens and yellows provide the phytochemicals lutein and zeaxanthin, compounds that are important for eye health and prevention of age-related macular degeneration, a leading cause of blindness in older people. These phytochemicals can be found in vegetables such as mustard greens, arugula, and summer squash. Many of us are taught that carrots are good for the eyes, and this is no misconception. Carrots and other orange fruits and vegetables are rich in alpha and beta carotene, precursors of vitamin A, which aid not only the eyes but the bones and immune system as well. The carotenes also function as antioxidants, cleansing free radicals from our bodies. Lastly, there are the red foods, for example, red peppers, tomatoes, and watermelons, which contain lycopene, a phytochemical which may help protect against breast cancer. [1]

As you browse the recipes of this chapter, allow your imagination to run wild. These recipes are merely suggestions that can be molded to your specific needs and taste buds. Pay notice to the colors of the ingredients used, with their aforementioned health benefits in mind. My hope is that you gain a sense of simplicity, beauty, and finesse for your healthy eating and cooking journey. If one solely focuses on health and pleasing our physiology, it can be easy to negate that which is also both pleasing to the eye and to our taste buds. However, we can, quite literally, have our cake and eat it too.

THANK YOU

Thank you, God, for showing me the way, holding me in your arms, and loving me as you do. Because of You all things are possible. I am so blessed and unbelievably grateful to be on this journey and to walk with You each day.

Thank you, Mom and Dad, for your unconditional love, support, and guidance. God truly blessed me with you as parents, and words cannot express my gratitude. I will always be your little girl. Thank you, Joey. You inspire me every day. I love you so much and am so proud to be your big sister.

To Leo: I love you so much! Thank you for always being there for me and for loving me unconditionally. And to my family, friends, and loved ones: Thank you for your love, presence, and support. You pick me up when I am down and further my sparkle when I am already shining. My heart is so full with you in my life.

~Samantha Cifelli

Lunch

By Samantha Cifelli

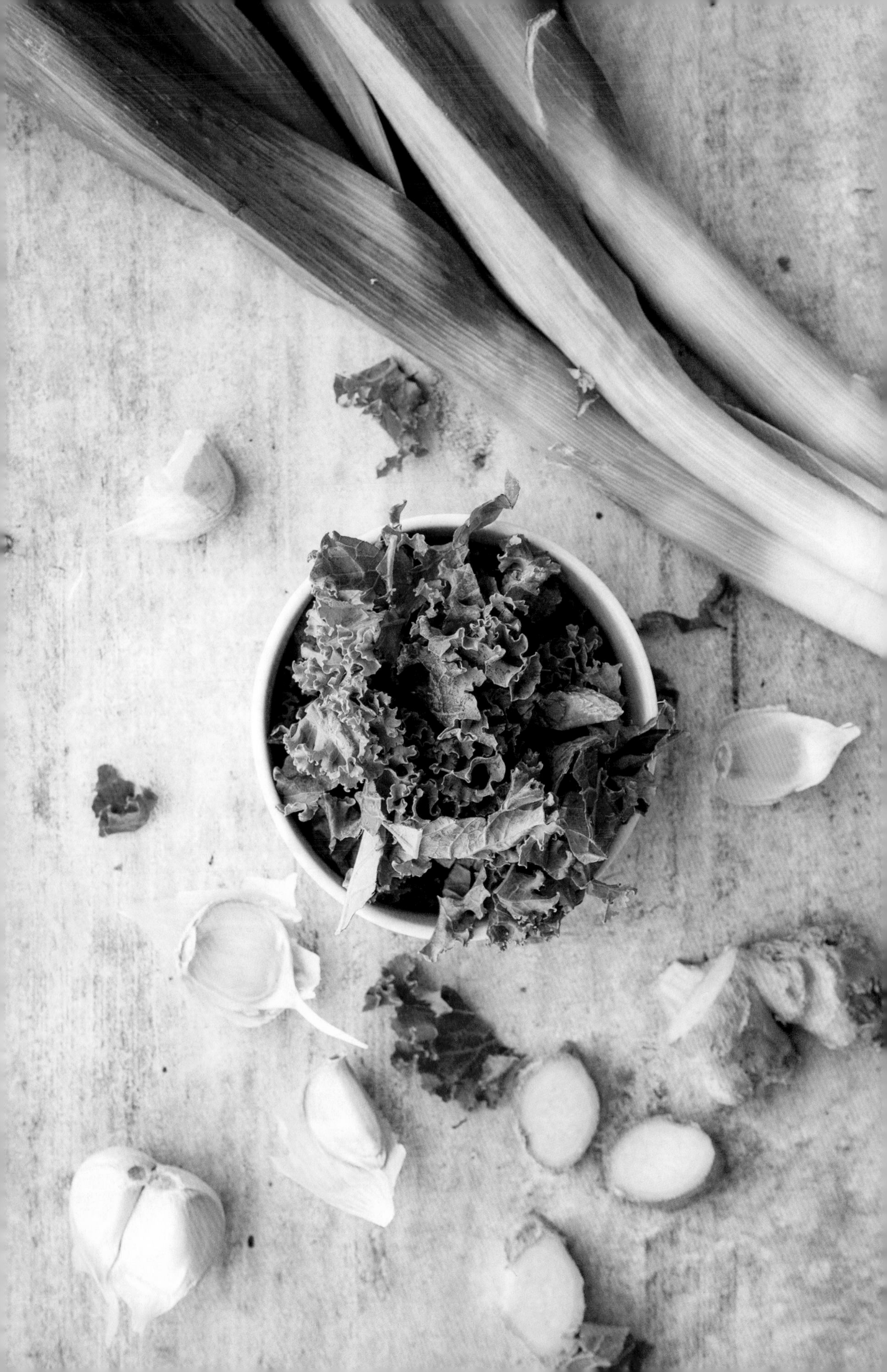

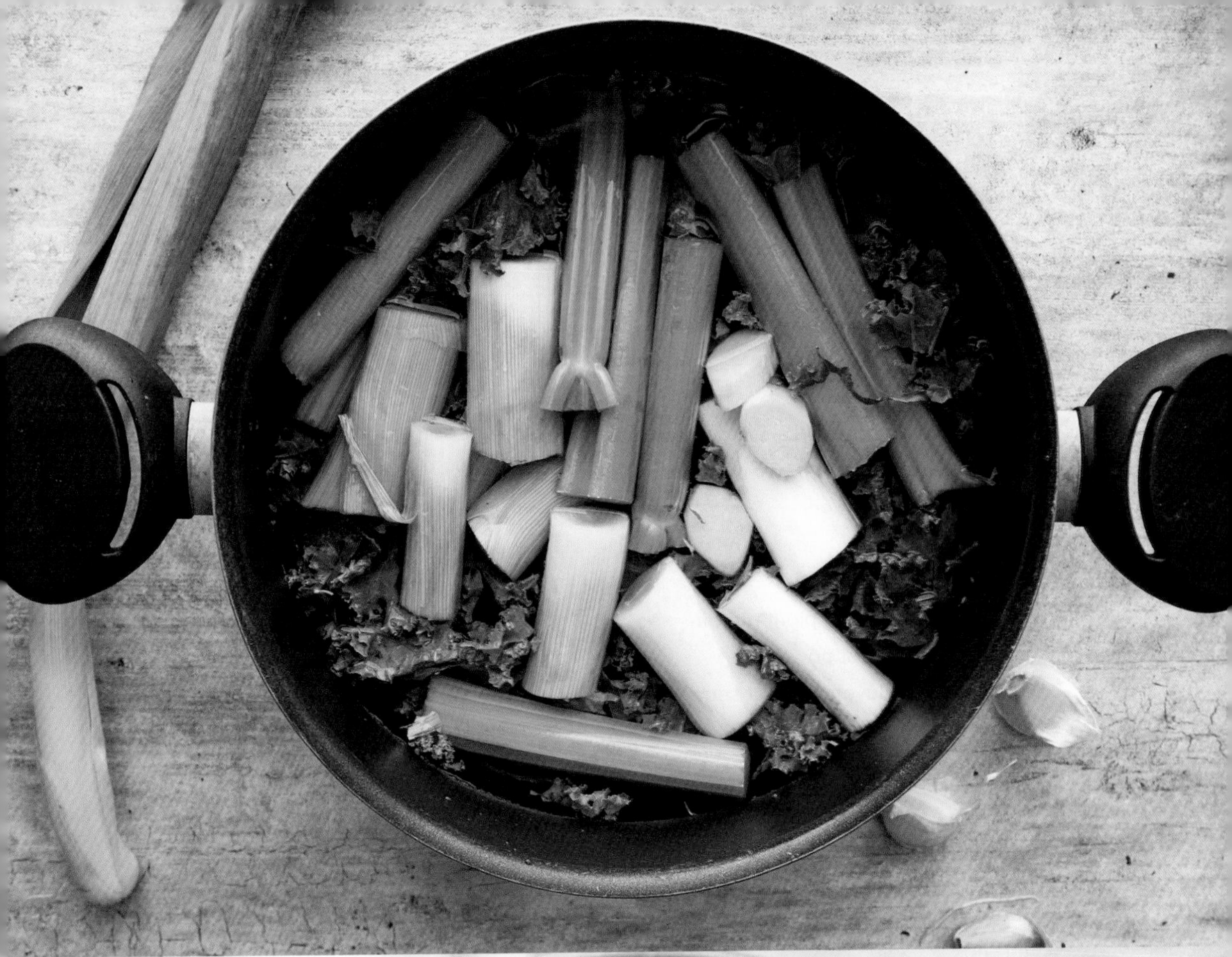
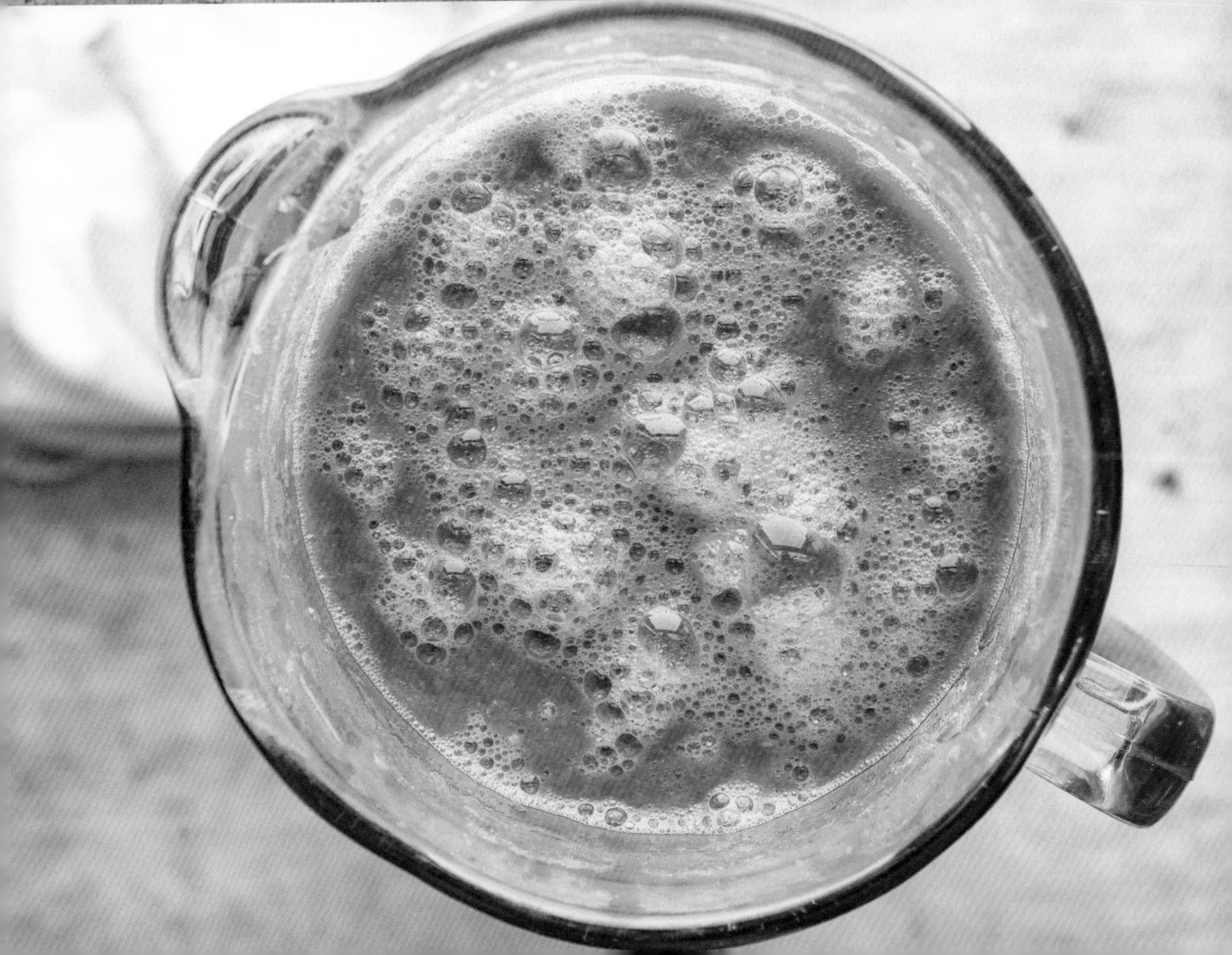

Eat Your Greens Soup

PREP TIME **15 minutes**
COOK TIME **20 minutes**
TOTAL TIME **35 minutes**

Ingredients

4 cups baby or regular kale

3 leeks, green tops and roots removed, chopped in half

4 pieces of celery, trimmed and chopped in half

3 tablespoons fresh ginger

4 cloves garlic

1 tablespoon cilantro

1 tablespoon unflavored plant protein

½ teaspoon maca root powder

2 teaspoons Himalayan or other sea salt

1 teaspoon black pepper

1 tablespoon extra virgin olive oil

½ cup coconut cream

Directions

1. Place kale, leeks, celery, and ginger in large pot, and fill with water, approximately ten cups.
2. Bring to boil, and continue to cook for ten minutes.
3. Strain liquid and reserve.
4. Place vegetables, ginger, about two cups of strained liquid, with garlic and cilantro into blender.
5. Blend until almost smooth.
6. Pour contents back into large pot.
7. Add plant protein, maca, sea salt, and pepper, and stir.
8. Stir in olive oil and coconut cream.
9. Bring soup to a simmer, and then turn off heat. Serve hot.

Happy Hormone Helpers

Kale is an excellent source of fiber, vitamins A, K, B6, and C, and minerals: manganese, copper, and calcium. Kale can assist in aiding mood swings, painful cramping, and bloating and can prevent bone degeneration. [2, 3]

Maca is a superfood known for its influence on hormonal balance. Maca is a great source of calcium, potassium, iron, fiber, and protein. It works by regulating the hypothalamus and pituitary glands in the brain, which can assist with hot flashes, low libido, and premenstrual syndrome.

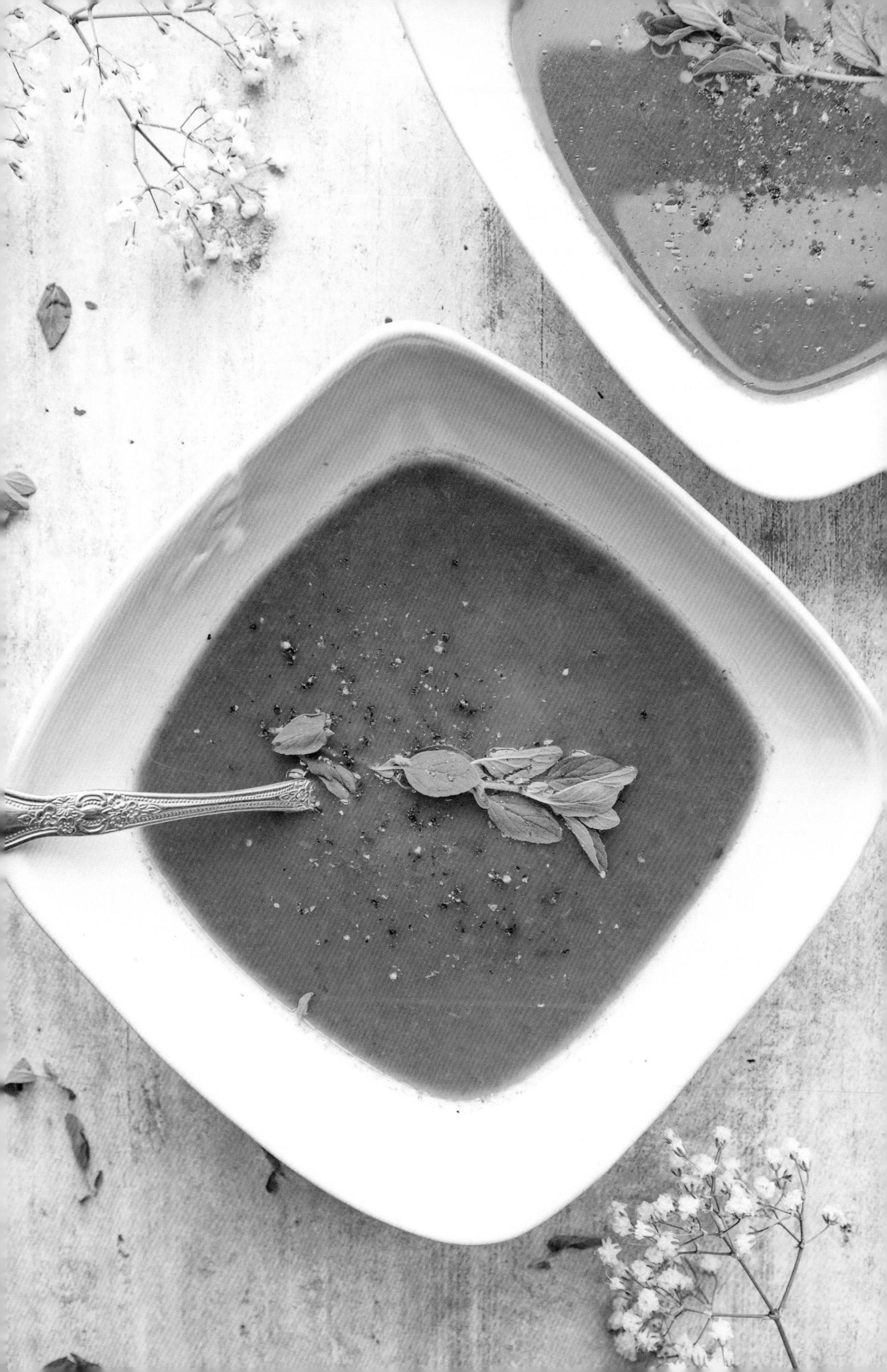

Super Greens and Pineapple Salad with Raspberry-Lemon Vinaigrette

PREP TIME **15 minutes**
COOK TIME **25 minutes**
TOTAL TIME **35 minutes**

Ingredients

1 cup Swiss chard

1 cup spinach

1 cup kale

1 fresh pineapple, diced

½ red pepper, diced

⅓ cup walnuts, chopped

¼ cup quinoa

⅓ cup wheatberries

Raspberry-lemon vinaigrette

Directions

1. Cook quinoa according to directions, and set aside to cool.

2. Mix Swiss chard, spinach, and kale in large bowl.

3. Toss in pineapple, red pepper, walnuts, and wheatberries.

4. Drizzle desired amount of raspberry-lemon vinaigrette over salad, and gently mix together.

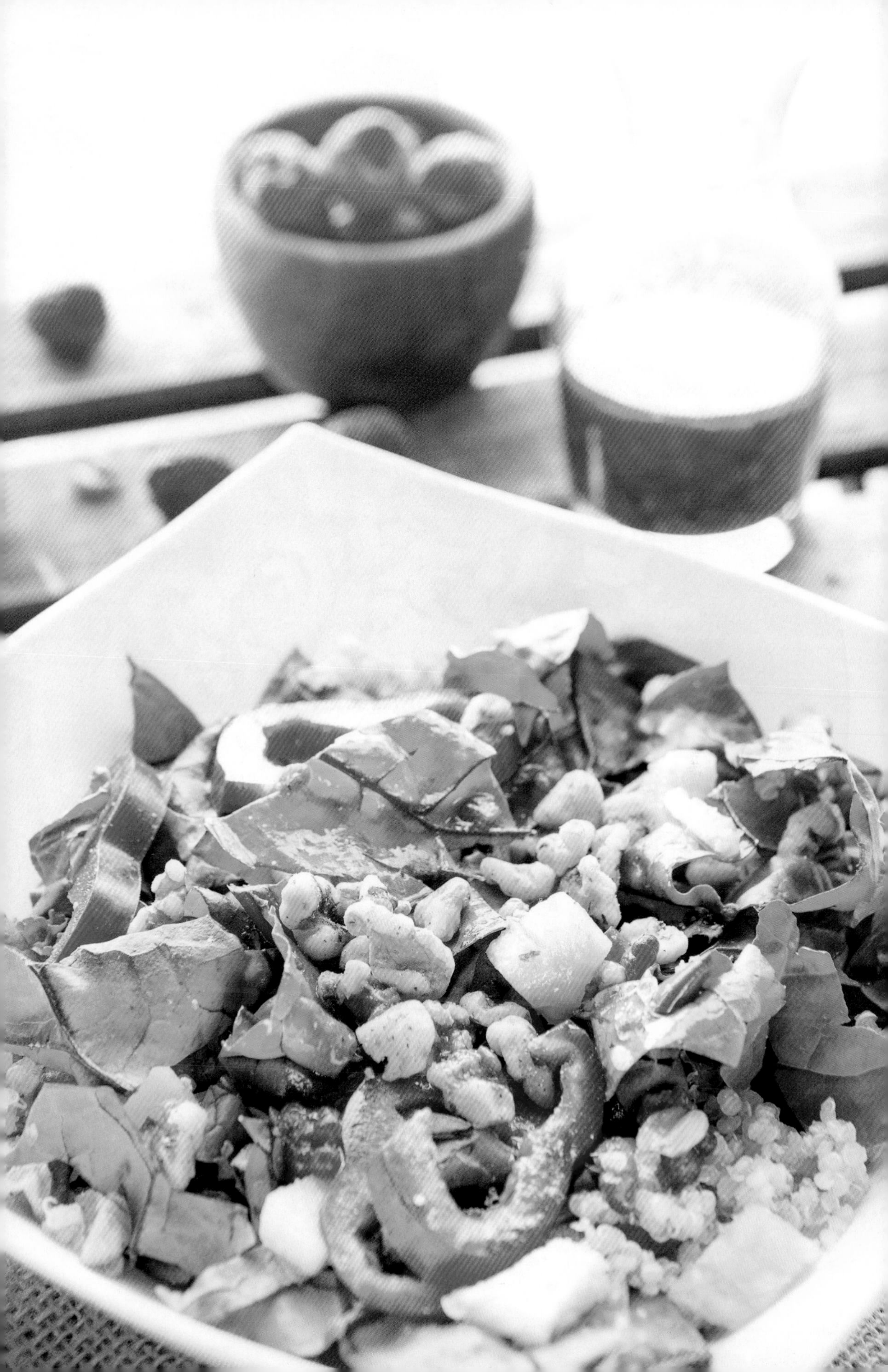

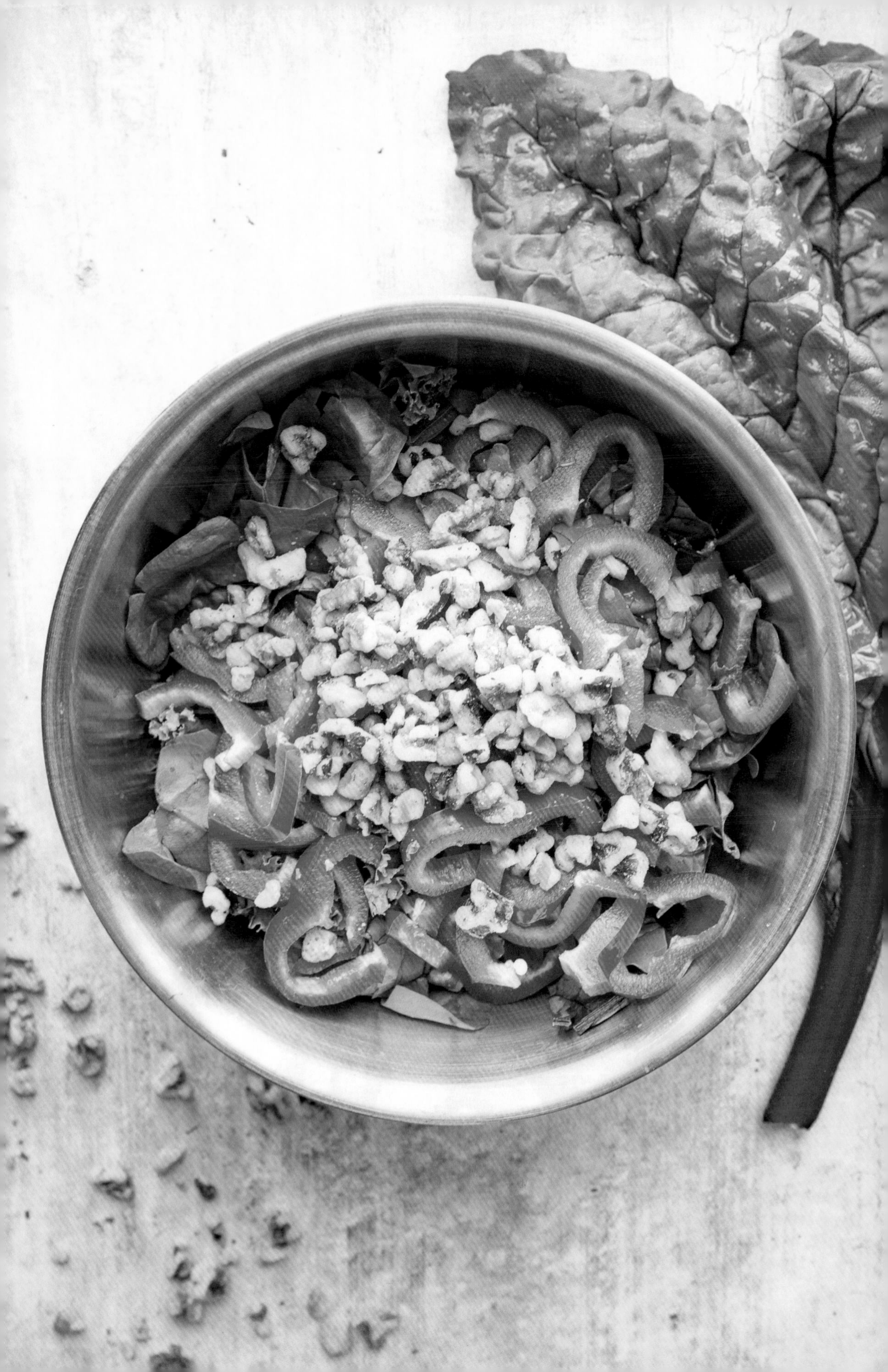

Raspberry-Lemon Vinaigrette

PREP TIME **1 minute**

Ingredients

½ cup raspberries

¼ cup extra virgin olive oil

¼ cup apple cider vinegar

2 tablespoons lemon juice (usually the juice of one lemon)

1 teaspoon Himalayan sea salt

Directions

1. Muddle raspberries in a small to medium bowl.
2. Slowly add in olive oil, then apple cider vinegar, whisking together with raspberries as you pour.
3. Add in lemon juice and salt, and whisk together.
4. Vinaigrette can be stored for up to four days in an airtight container in the refrigerator.

Happy Hormone Helpers

Walnuts are rich in phytosterols, known cancer fighters, as well as heart and bone friendly omega-3 fatty acids.[3]

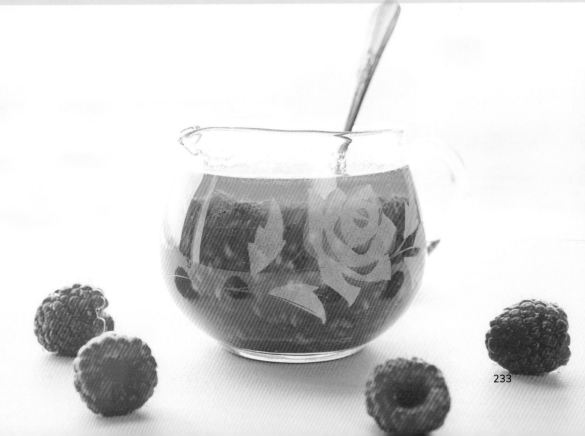

233

Whole Wheat Vegetable Pita with Sunflower Garlic Spread

PREP TIME **15 minutes**

Ingredients

1 whole wheat pita, sliced open—can substitute for gluten-free wrap, bread, or pita if gluten-free

3 tablespoons sunflower garlic spread

4 slices avocado

3 slices tomato

3 slices cucumber

½ carrot, shredded

1 sliced red onion

Directions

1. Spread sunflower garlic spread on both sides of the inside of whole wheat pita

2. Stuff pita with avocado, tomato, cucumber, shredded carrot, and red onion.

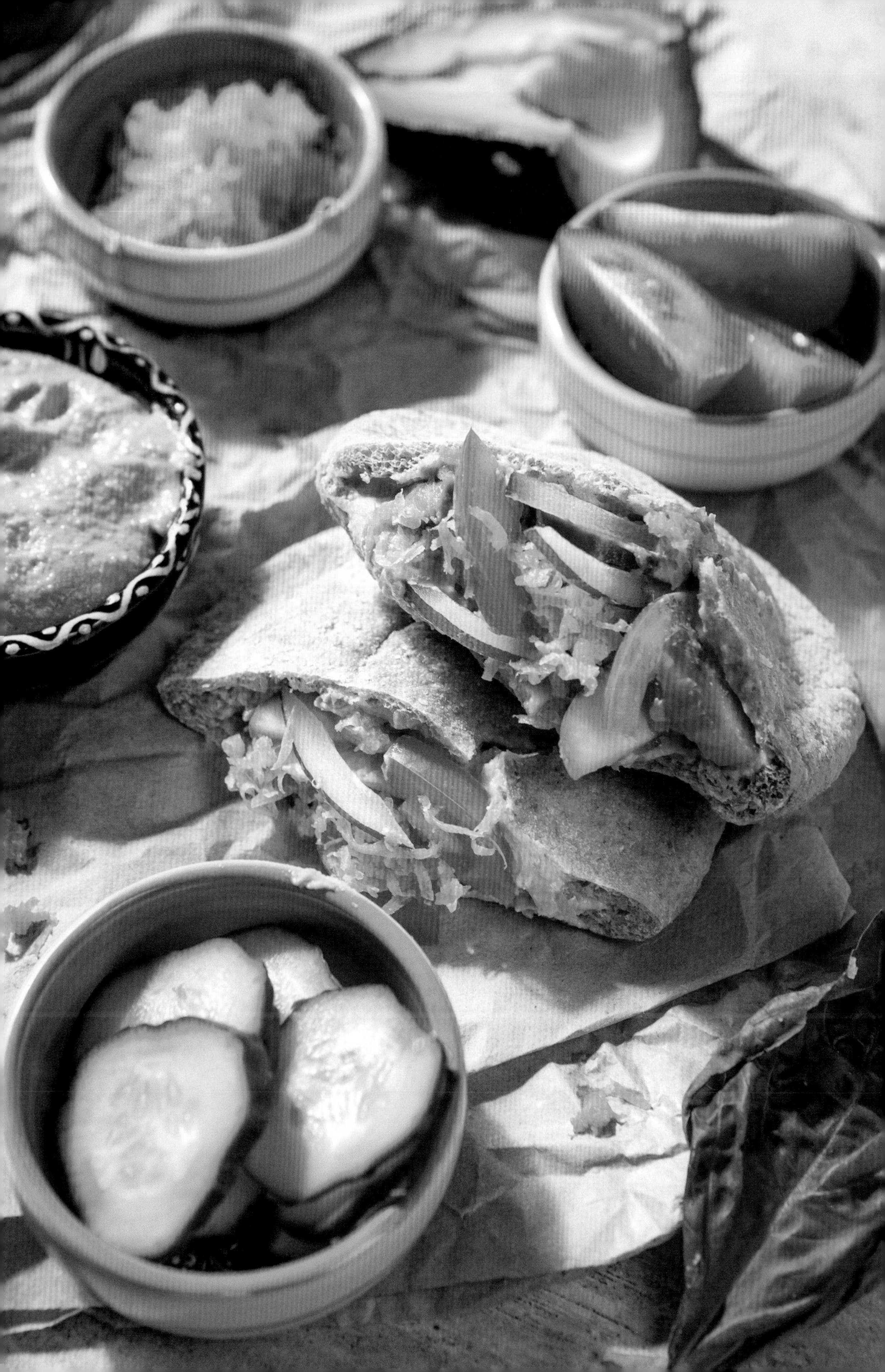

Sunflower Garlic Spread

PREP TIME **2 minutes**

Ingredients

1 cup raw sunflower seeds

8 cloves of garlic, diced

8 leaves of basil, fresh

¼ cup extra virgin olive oil

½ cup unsweetened almond milk

2 tablespoons lemon juice (usually the juice of one lemon)

1 teaspoon Himalayan sea salt, or more to taste

Directions

1. Add sunflower seeds to blender or food processor, and grind until powdered.

2. Add in garlic, basil, oil, milk, lemon juice, and salt, and pulse until a paste is formed.

3. Spread can be stored in refrigerator for one week.

Happy Hormone Helpers

Avocados are rich in monounsaturated fats, which are beneficial for hair, skin, and nail health. While bananas are known for their potassium content, avocados are an even better source of the mineral, beneficial for blood pressure control. [4]

Observational studies have shown that the lycopene in tomatoes may ward off breast and cervical cancers. Lycopene in tomatoes, combined with a heart healthy oil such as extra virgin olive oil, play a protective role against cardiovascular disease.[3]

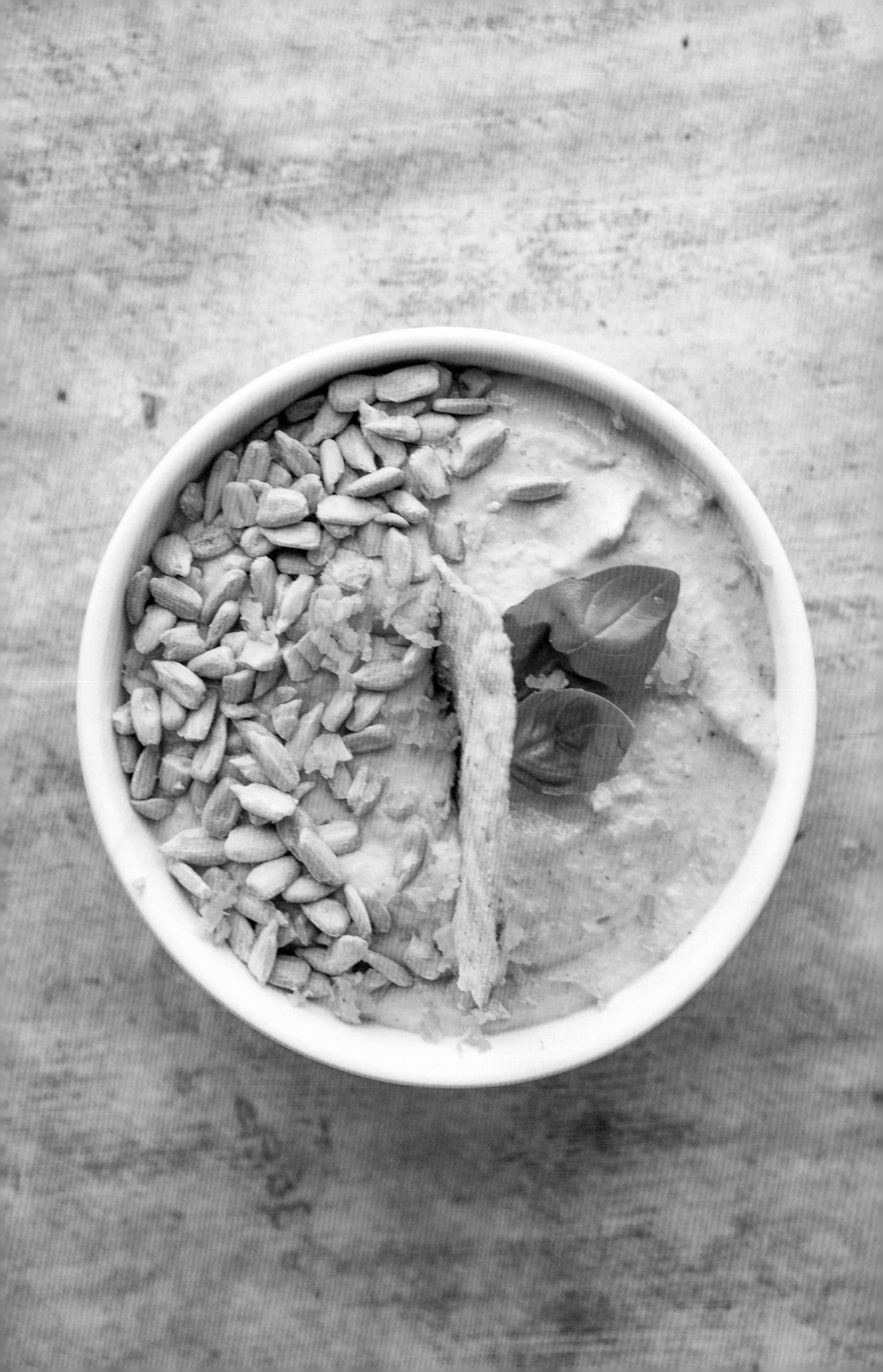

Pineapple, White Peach, And Arugula Pizzette On Quinoa Crust

PREP TIME 10 minutes
QUINOA CRUST PREP TIME
overnight or 8 hours
COOK TIME 40 minutes

Ingredients

Pizza Toppings

½ white peach, pitted and thinly sliced

5 spears of fresh pineapple

1 ½ cups fresh arugula

2 tablespoons balsamic glaze

Himalayan sea salt, to taste

Cracked black pepper, to taste

Quinoa Crust

¾ cup quinoa, rinsed and drained

¼ cup water

1 teaspoon baking powder

1 tablespoon extra virgin olive oil

Directions

Overnight:

1. Put quinoa in a bowl, and cover it with water.

2. Let the quinoa soak overnight or for at least eight hours.

Next Day:

1. Preheat oven to 425F.

2. Rinse and drain quinoa again.

3. In a food processor, put the quinoa, water, salt, and baking powder.

4. Process the mix for about two minutes or until smooth in consistency.

5. Line a 9 inch cake pan with parchment paper.

6. Pour oil over the parchment paper.

7. Pour the batter into the cake pan over the oil, and smooth it out evenly.

8. Bake the crust for 15 minutes.

9. Flip the crust, and bake for another 5 minutes.

Topping Directions

1. Keep oven at 425F.

2. On outdoor or indoor grill, grill pineapple spears on high heat for 2 to 3 minutes on each side, or until grill marks appear. Set aside.

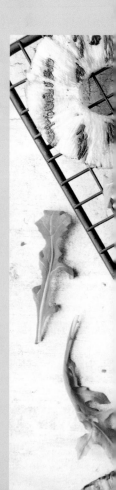

238

3. Place kneaded pizza dough on pizza stone or lightly oiled baking pan

Top dough liberally with arugula, peach, and pineapple slices, salt, and pepper.

4. Bake in oven for about 5 minutes.

5. Drizzle balsamic glaze over the pizzette.

6. Allow pizzette to cool.

7. Slice and serve.

Balsamic Glaze Ingredients

1 cup balsamic vinegar

Directions

1. Pour balsamic vinegar into a medium saucepan over medium heat.

2. Once boiling, reduce heat and simmer for 15 minutes or until thickened.

3. Use immediately, or store in airtight container once cooled.

Happy Hormone Helpers

Arugula or "rocket" is rich in vitamin K, crucial for bone health and calcium regulation.[5] Arugula and white peaches are both rich in vitamin C, a key micronutrient for skin health, helping to reduce the appearance of wrinkles and combat any environmentally caused skin damage. Vitamin C is also involved in collagen production.[5, 6]

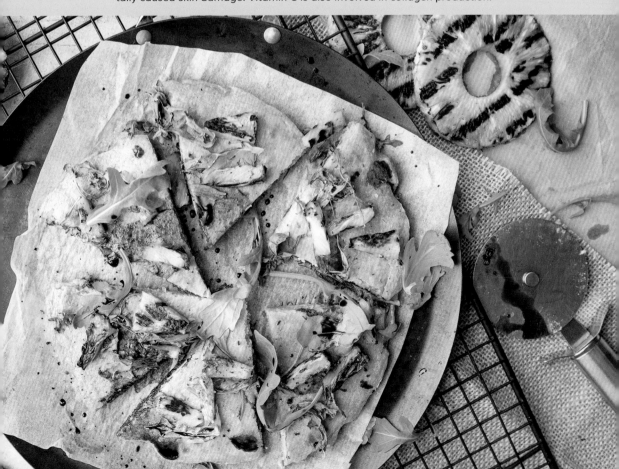

PLANTS ON PLATES: POSSIBILITIES, PASSION, A PATH, AND A PLAN

FOOD IS EVERYTHING. FOOD IS FAMILY. FOOD IS MEMORIES. FOOD IS MEDICINE. FOOD BRINGS US TOGETHER. FOOD KEEPS US TOGETHER.

By Margie Cook

Registered Holistic Nutritionist RHN
Certified Vegan Lifestyle Coach
Educator VLCE

Margie Cook

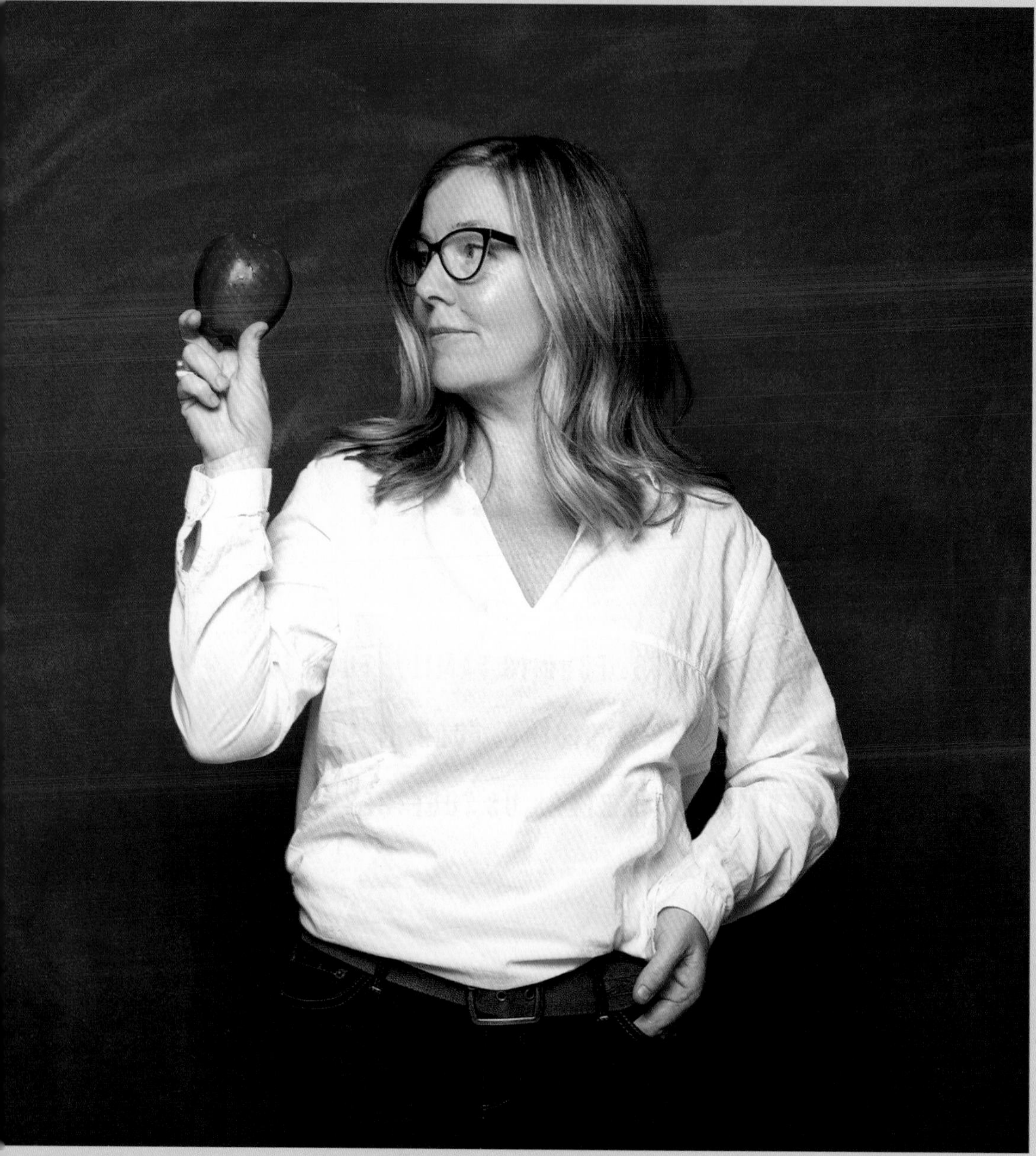

It's always been about food for Margie Cook. When she returned to school to become a registered holistic nutritionist (RHN) and a certified vegan lifestyle coach and educator (VLCE), it only made sense that her focus would become plant-based cooking, eating and educating.

Margie's vegetarianism began in her early twenties, but her road to veganism was a colorful journey that played out over many years. Margie genuinely loves people, and because of that she genuinely wants everyone to live the happiest life possible. Through extensive research, contemplation and experimentation, she realized that when it comes to food, health and happiness, you can't have one without the other. "Food is joyful," she explains, "It's about laughter, family, and feeling good about yourself."

Always one to experiment in the kitchen, this new enlightenment brought on a passion fueled by a desire to discover and create delicious, filling and beautiful plant-based recipes that could stand up to even the most skeptical omnivore. Margie's love of, and innate sense of flavor, her exceptional palate, skill and spark for life has helped her design plant-based foods that are both tantalizing and sublime. She believes every meal you eat is a chance to take a step towards better self awareness, glowing skin, more energy, and a healthier planet. Through customized cooking classes, corporate wellness programs and coaching, along with recipe development and restaurant menu consulting, catering and personal chef services, Margie brings her unique, lighthearted style to the hearts and minds (and tables) of all she meets. "My goal is never short-term," she says. "I want to act as a guide to a heightened understanding of the joys and benefits of a plant-based lifestyle."

Margie lives in Streetsville, Ontario just outside of her hometown Toronto, with her husband, four kids, and their big yellow dog.

WWW.MARGIEC OOK.COM | WWW.PLANTSONPLATES.COM
ig: _plantsonplates | fb: Plants On Plates

If something around diet and nutrition sounds too good to be true, with very few exceptions, it is. Just when you think you've got it all figured out, along comes another headline or study, convincingly stating the exact opposite of what you just finished getting your head around. All these conflicting messages around our health and food choices are dizzying and confusing and in many cases, make us feel like no matter what we do today, it simply won't apply tomorrow, so why bother?

There is no such thing as a magic pill or quick fix, so the sooner we learn to be our own guides and stop buying into short term, one size fits all, often expensive band aid solutions the better. Doing so, only prolongs getting to the real work of feeding ourselves while acknowledging and trying to mend our broken, inequitable, and inherently cruel food system. Nothing in life that is worthwhile is easy, not at first anyway. An indisputable and incredibly hopeful thought though is this: we all have the opportunity, every single day, to write our personal prescription for health. This begins and ends with things like our thoughts, who we surround ourselves with, how we choose to serve this world, and how often we move our bodies, but ultimately, health and longevity is more often than not decided by what we put on

"Genetics loads the gun, lifestyle pulls the trigger."
~ CALDWELL B. ESSELSTYN, JR., MD, CLEVELAND CLINIC

our plates and into our mouths. We truly are what we eat, so listen to your gut.

This is not an all or nothing world and what works for one may not work for another. Eating the way that makes you feel happy and supported is the key to long term success. If you feel like you have tried just about everything out there in the *diet* department, as did I, except an all or mostly plant-based one, then this is your lucky day. What could you possibly have to lose by adding in more plant food and lightening your karmic and environmental load in the process? Plants on Plates checks every box on our collective *what can little old me do to help save the planet* list, and the *I can't possibly make a difference to all that is broken and backward in our food system all by myself* mindset. Oh yes you can! This is outdated thinking and thoughts like these are holding us back. If we all consciously swap out animal based ingredients on a daily, weekly, or monthly basis, Plants on Plates becomes the new normal and together we can make a tremendous difference. Together we start a movement. Individuals have power when they band together and grassroots movements are at the heart of all social change. When we buck the norm and swim upstream against all the processed and chemical dripping fast food and skip the packaging and the endocrine disrupting plastics to choose whole, plant foods instead, we make a statement and we take back some power from industries that most definitely do not have the best interest of anything in mind except their bottom line. [1] If we all start voting with our grocery dollars, change will come. And it must. The clock is ticking.

People choose plant-based diets for a multitude of reasons, all of them are compelling and all slightly different in their flavor and color. With everything we understand about the destructive nature of animal agriculture these days, it is becoming increasingly difficult to be an environmentalist and consume animals. There is also very strong evidence that indicates a whole-food plant-based diet can prevent and sometimes even reverse some chronic diseases.

Some incredible documentaries to watch on the benefits of a plant-based diet are *Cowspiracy* for the planet and *Forks over Knives* for real life stories about what happens when people choose food as medicine.

When my second husband and I first met and began eating together, he started to notice changes in his body which at first seemed impossible for him to believe until undeniable patterns began to emerge. Both of us being single parents every other week meant that we had a very set dating pattern for the first year until our kids met: together for one week and then off the next week, as we parented in separate cities. The weeks we were together and he ate plant-based meals with me, his digestion improved, aches and pains he had put down to what he assumed was a genetic guarantee (arthritis) all but disappeared, he slept better and his skin glowed, yet within twenty-four hours of going back to *his* way, all these symptoms came rushing back in, week after week. Symptoms are the only way our bodies have of letting us know something is wrong. Fatigue, bloating, aches and pains, headaches, congestion, acne, restlessness, irritability, these are all symptoms, and yet our inclination is to normalize them rather than drill deeper and figure out their root cause. We tend to accept them as a right of passage, a normal part of whatever stage of life we currently reside in, take a pill, and move on. We think, "Well, my mom had arthritis, so I guess I do too," or, "Grandma had high blood pressure, so is it is any wonder I do as well?"

This way of thinking is outdated and seriously, if we don't carve out time for our personal health right now, then what is the point of any of it? What is the point of achieving success now if we are not healthy enough to enjoy it down the road? Think long term. Think long term about the planet and our own bodies (and the animals— please always remember and seriously consider the animals). Think about how long we want to live, and I am not simply referring to throwing out a big number. Consider quality over quantity. If we are already experiencing symptoms that are affecting our ability to live the way we wish we could, then wouldn't it behoove us to forecast a few more years or decades, and try and imagine how we might feel then if our current state is already slightly compromised? If there were something that could be done today that would almost guarantee feeling better tomorrow and for years to come, is there a downside to trying? The future will be much brighter if we can let go of outdated ideas and models that aren't serving anyone anymore and stop clinging to them as though they are life rafts, when in fact, they are the sinking ship. We are talking about consciously swapping out animal based ingredients as often as possible and replacing them, without any compromise with delicious plant-based alternatives.

When transitioning to a more plant-based diet we need to prepare. Make reclaiming your kitchen your new Netflix for a few months (or watch Netflix while you prepare yummy food!). Spend a few hours every weekend planning your week of whole food eating, then shop, and do some prep. You cannot go wrong when you can open the fridge and have delicious options at your fingertips, greens washed, veggies chopped and, you guessed it, a plan. And remember, it isn't the animal or animal product that we crave, but rather the comfort and the satiation we experience from familiar textures and flavors. Textures and flavors that are woven into our DNA, into our memories, into our histories. Textures and flavors that are readily available in the plant kingdom with a little imagination and rewiring. Don't *give something up*, add something in instead and honestly let your body decide. A magical thing happens when we fuel our bodies with more plants. They have this way of gently elbowing out things we have been consuming that no longer serve us. As Victor Hugo so eloquently said, "There is nothing more powerful than an idea whose time has come." I couldn't agree more. The power of plants is indisputable.

THANK YOU

Thanks to all the little birds, shafts of sunlight, and lazy rivers that keep me on and off my path following their songs, basking in their promise and floating in their currents and of course to my family and friends for always believing in me...no matter what.

~ Margie Cook

Dinner

By Margie Cook

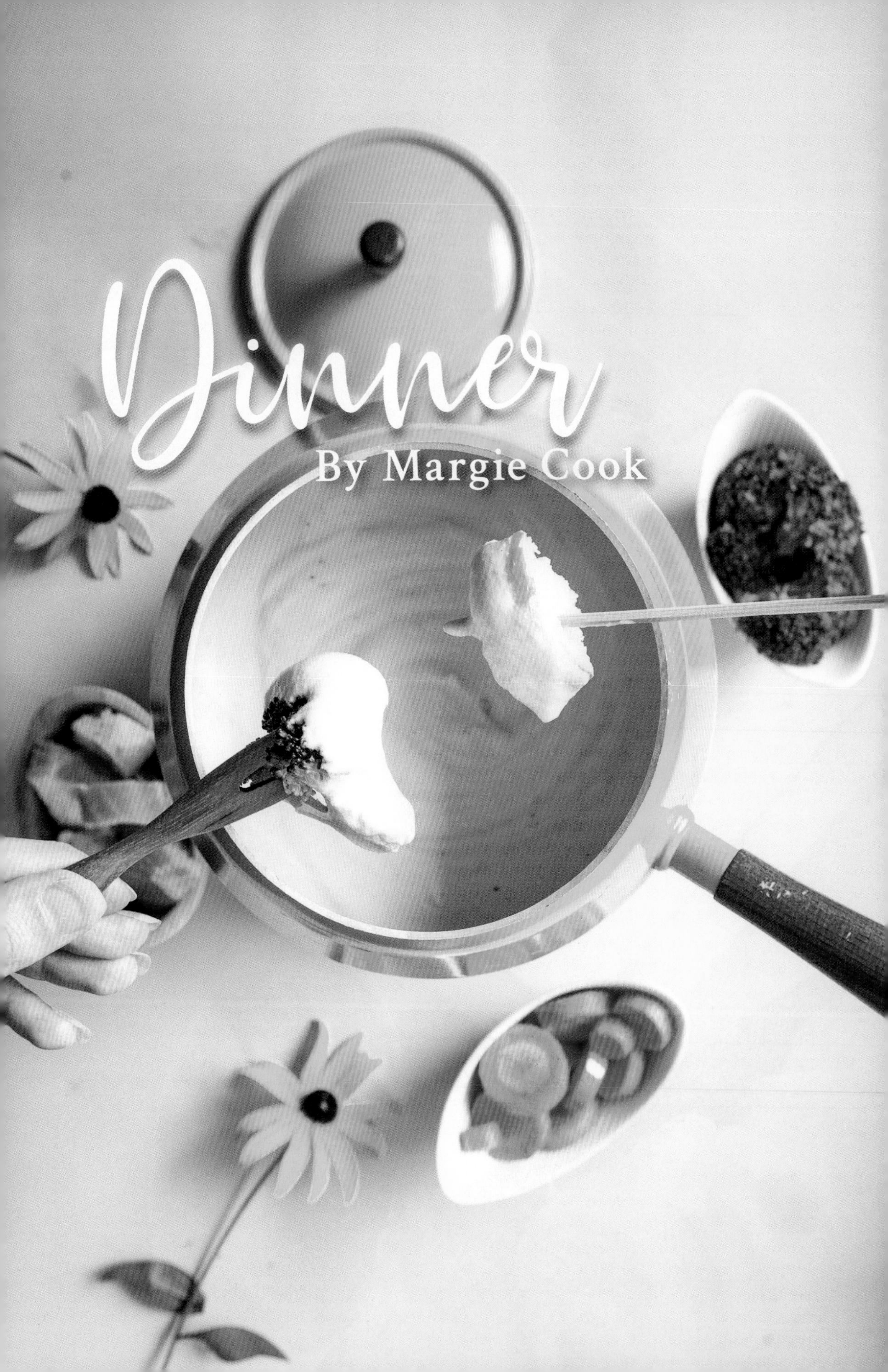

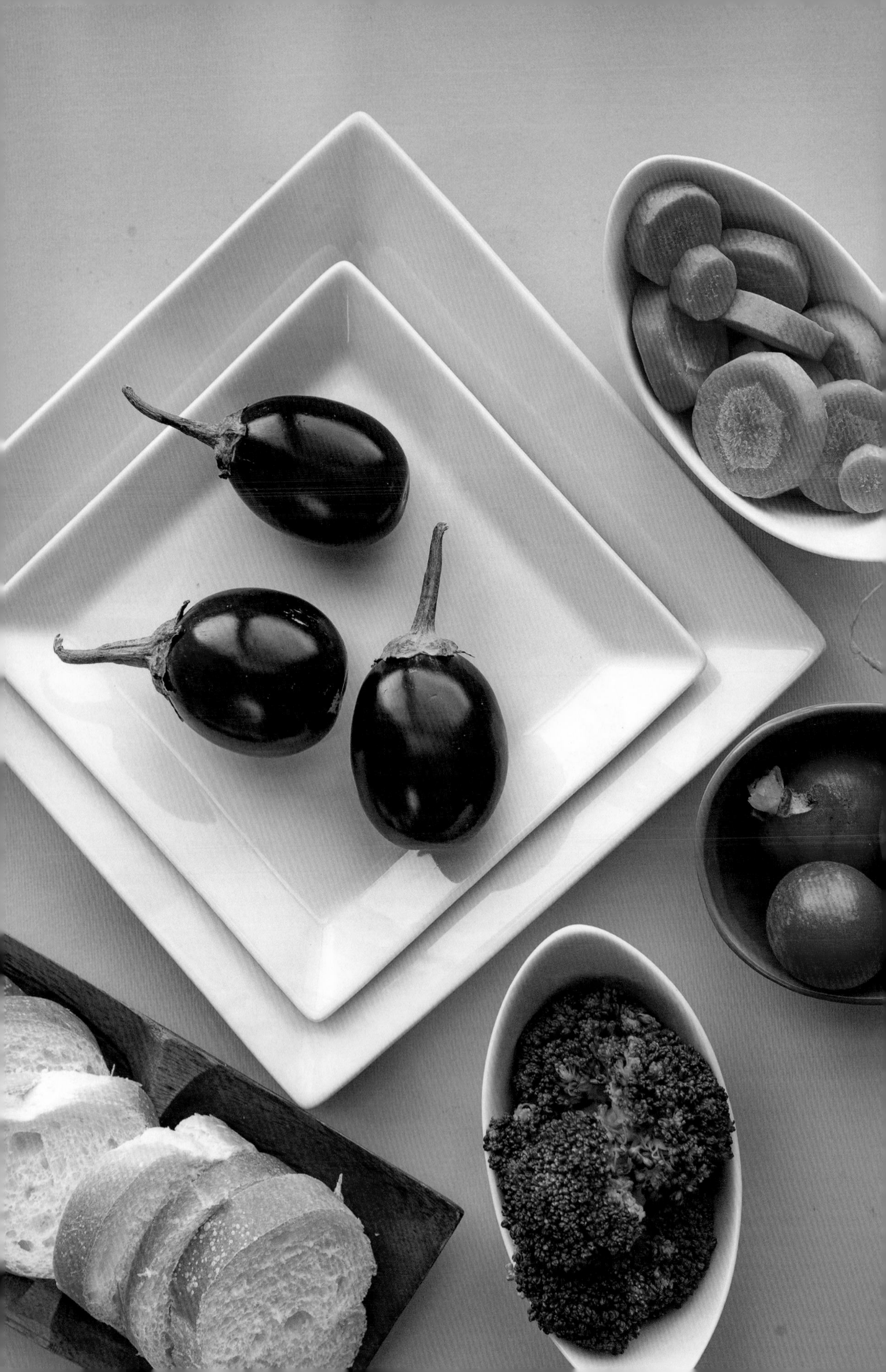

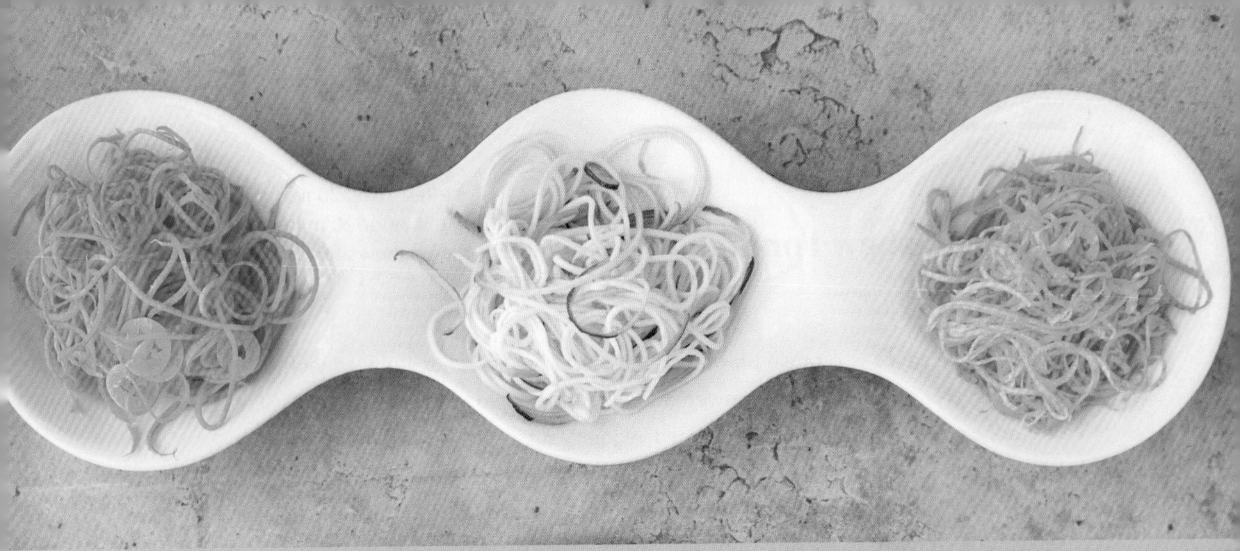

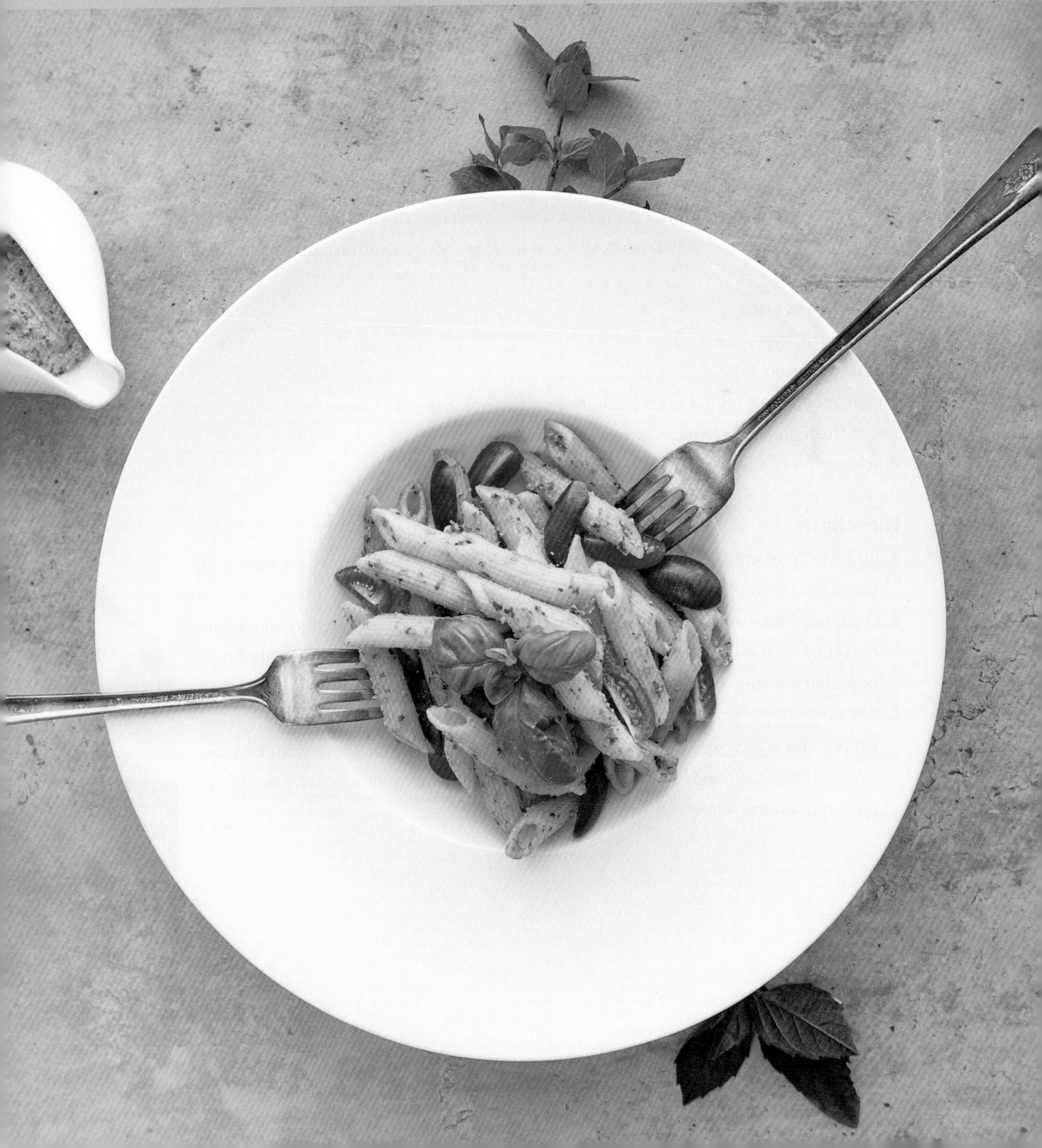

Garlic Cashew Fondue

PREP TIME 20 minutes
TOTAL PREP TIME 1 hour 20 minutes -
includes soaking the cashews for an hour

This versatile sauce is a mash up of many different recipes I have played with over the years. It is perfect for plant-powered fondue fun served with crusty bread (GF if desired) and either raw or lightly steamed veggies, but it doesn't end there! Try it on a roasted or steamed vegetable side dish, potatoes, or pasta (think Fettuccini Alfredo minus the regret and food coma). I can literally think of fifty ways to use this cheese sauce. It is stunning in its simplicity and deliciousness! Cashews are magical. You'll see.

Ingredients

2 cups water

⅔ cup dry white wine (always cook with a wine you would drink!)

or

¼ cup raw organic apple cider (tangy) or unseasoned rice vinegar (mellow)

¾ cup raw, unsalted cashews- soaked for at least an hour to soften- drain and rinse

3 large cloves garlic

⅓ cup nutritional yeast

2 teaspoons sea salt

1 tablespoon fresh lemon juice (omit if using vinegar instead of wine)

⅓ cup fresh parsley- stir in or sprinkle on top

Black pepper to taste

Directions

1. Add all ingredients up to and including lemon juice into a high-speed blender and blend until smooth.

2. Once the sauce gains a milky consistency in the blender, pour it into a saucepan and cook over medium heat, whisking constantly to avoid sticking. It will bubble, pop, and amaze you as it thickens. Approximately 10 minutes.

3. Stir in the fresh parsley and pepper at this point and pour into fondue pot or simply into a warmed bowl in the middle of the table. Individual ramekins on dinner plates surrounded by bread and veggies for dipping makes for a beautiful presentation as well.

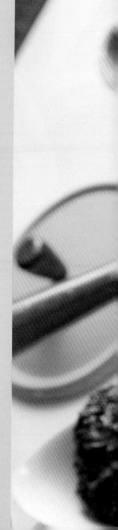

Happy Hormone Helpers

Nutritional Yeast (affectionately called nooch) is an inactive yeast and a great source of B vitamins (including B12, but it would be fortified with it not naturally occurring), an important supplement for vegans). It is super cheesy and delicious so vegans love to sprinkle it on just about anything (even POPCORN!). Combined with hemp seeds, garlic powder, and sea salt, it makes a divine stand in for parmesan cheese.

Cashews contain plenty of zinc, a mineral which plays an important role in hormone production.

Apple Cider Vinegar has a myriad of health benefits associated with it. Choose organic, raw and unfiltered vinegar containing the health benefits of mother (the live fermentation, the cloudy sediment in the bottle that has small amounts of fiber, amino acids, enzymes and loads of good probiotic bacteria). A shot a day helps the body convert proteins into amino acids which are responsible for the creation of our hormones, balancing blood sugar levels and maintaining healthy pH levels in the body, thus helping good bacteria flourish.

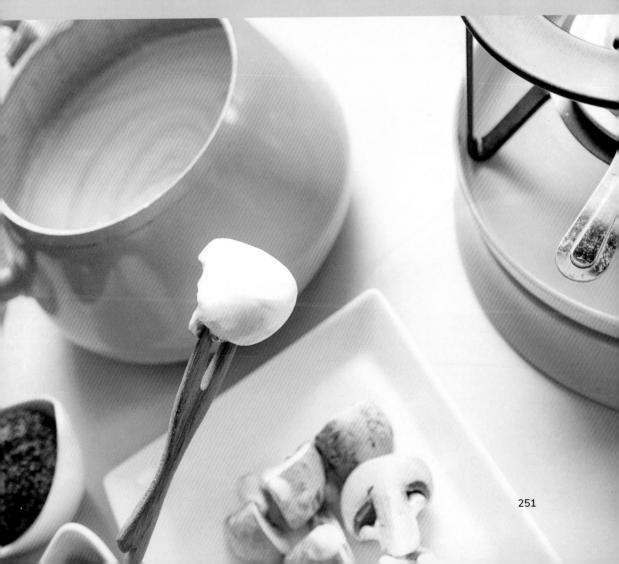

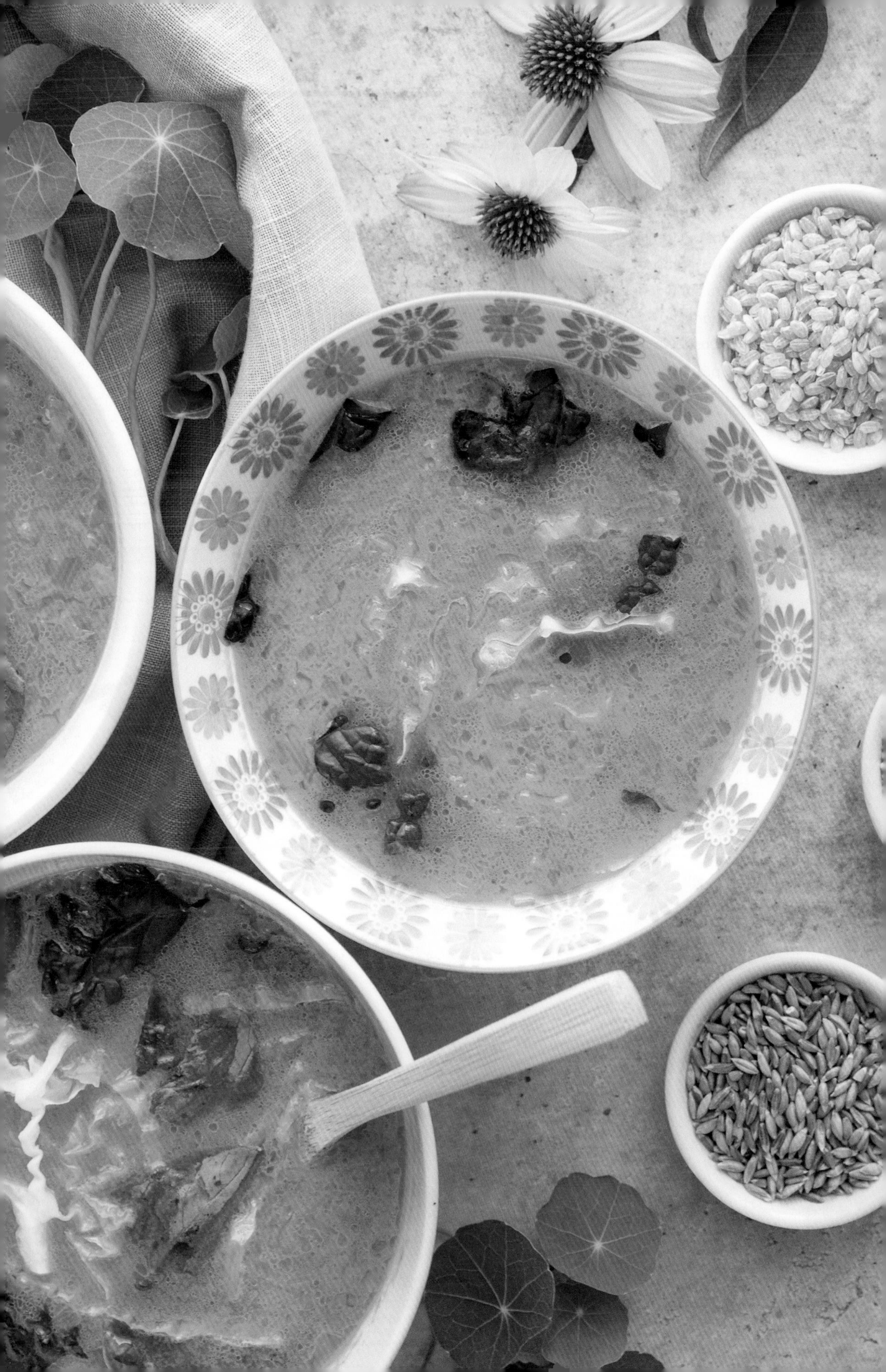

PREP TIME 30 minutes
COOK TIME 90 minutes - includes 1
hour of recommended simmering
TOTAL TIME 110 minutes

Magic Mushroom Soup

Move over chicken soup and a hip check to you, cheesy French onion, because the ingredients in this fully plant-powered soup are truly magical and blissfully soul soothing, no matter what the weather is doing outside. Make on a chilly winter's night, on a rainy day at the lake, or during a heat wave in July. Seriously make this soup anytime because these immune boosting, superhero ingredients will massage you into soup submission and leave you and your cells ready for battle... or a good book. If extra hungry, stir in cooked brown rice, quinoa, or farro—but then you must call it Magic Mushroom Stewp instead!

Ingredients

1-2 tablespoons avocado oil

1 large yellow or white onion, chopped (approximately 2 cups)

4 scallions—white only, thinly sliced— (see below for green ends)

5 garlic cloves—chopped (2 generous tablespoons)

2 tablespoons fresh ginger—finely minced—no need to peel if organic, just wash

4 celery stalks—chopped (approximately 2 cups)

5 large Portobello mushrooms (approximately 6 cups)

2 cups Napa cabbage (or cabbage of choice)—shredded or chopped

2 tablespoons tamari

1 tablespoon ground turmeric

2 teaspoons Himalayan pink salt or sea salt

5 cups water

1(400ml) can coconut milk (full fat)

3 heads baby bok choy—chopped (approximately 4 cups loosely packed)

1 bunch kale, remove stem and chop (approximately 2 cups)

4 scallions—green half —chopped into rounds

Fresh baby spinach to line soup bowls—chop or leave leaves whole

Some hot pepper flakes to garnish (optional)

Serve with a wedge of lime to squeeze over top, fresh black pepper, and sea salt.

Directions

1. Chop onion and scallions (set aside green end of the scallions for later).

2. Mince garlic and ginger, chop celery and dice mushrooms into uniform pieces. Shred or roughly chop cabbage.

3. Heat oil in a large soup pot over medium heat.

4. Add onions and white ends of scallions and sauté for a few minutes. Add garlic and ginger and cook for a few more minutes. Stirring.

5. Add celery, mushrooms, and cabbage to the pot and sauté for 5–10 minutes.

6. Add the tamari, turmeric, sea salt, water, and coconut milk, and bring to a gentle boil.

7. Turn down heat and lightly simmer, covered, for at least an hour. Stirring occasionally.

8. After chopping, washing and spinning dry, add the kale and baby bok choy 5–10 minutes before serving. Warm the greens, but try not to cook them. Add scallion greens at the very last minute.

9. If not serving immediately, let soup cool on stovetop and store in the refrigerator. When ready to serve, re-heat and add the kale, bok choy, and scallions.

10. Line soup bowls or soup plates with fresh spinach for an extra punch of greens, and ladle soup over top. Sprinkle with optional hot pepper flakes, extra grated ginger, and sesame seeds. Serve with a wedge of fresh lime.

11. Soup will keep for several days in the fridge... but it won't last that long since it's oh so delicious!

Happy Hormone Helpers

Avocado Oil has a similar nutritional makeup to olive oil, with the added benefits of being a source of bioavailable phyto-testosterone, having anti-estrogenic properties to prevent estrogen excess, and containing fats your hormones need to be transported around your bloodstream. How cool is that?

Mushrooms are the best vegetable source of vitamin D!

Garlic is in a league of its own. As if being an antioxidant and anti-inflammatory weren't enough, garlic, **onions**, chives, **scallions,** and shallots to a lesser extent contain amazingly high concentrations of the compound allicin which improves the body's ability to metabolize iron, an important part of balancing hormones. Yes please!

Napa Cabbage cruciferous vegetables = happy hormones

Turmeric is a "golden herb" in Ayurveda due to its antioxidant, anti-microbial, and anti-inflammatory properties. Turmeric has proven estrogenic activity which means it mimics the activity of the hormone. Curcumin acts as a phytoestrogen (which is estrogen from a plant source). This could explain why it is so useful in female reproductive health.

Himalayan Pink Salt The more we add this show-off-ski natural salt with its 84 different trace minerals to our hormone-healthy diet, the better!

Bok Choy packed with vitamin C and K: don't underestimate this vegetable!

Kale and other dark leafy greens, like **spinach** and **bok choy** provide the body with a boost of natural magnesium, iron, and zinc which are all necessary for hormone health.

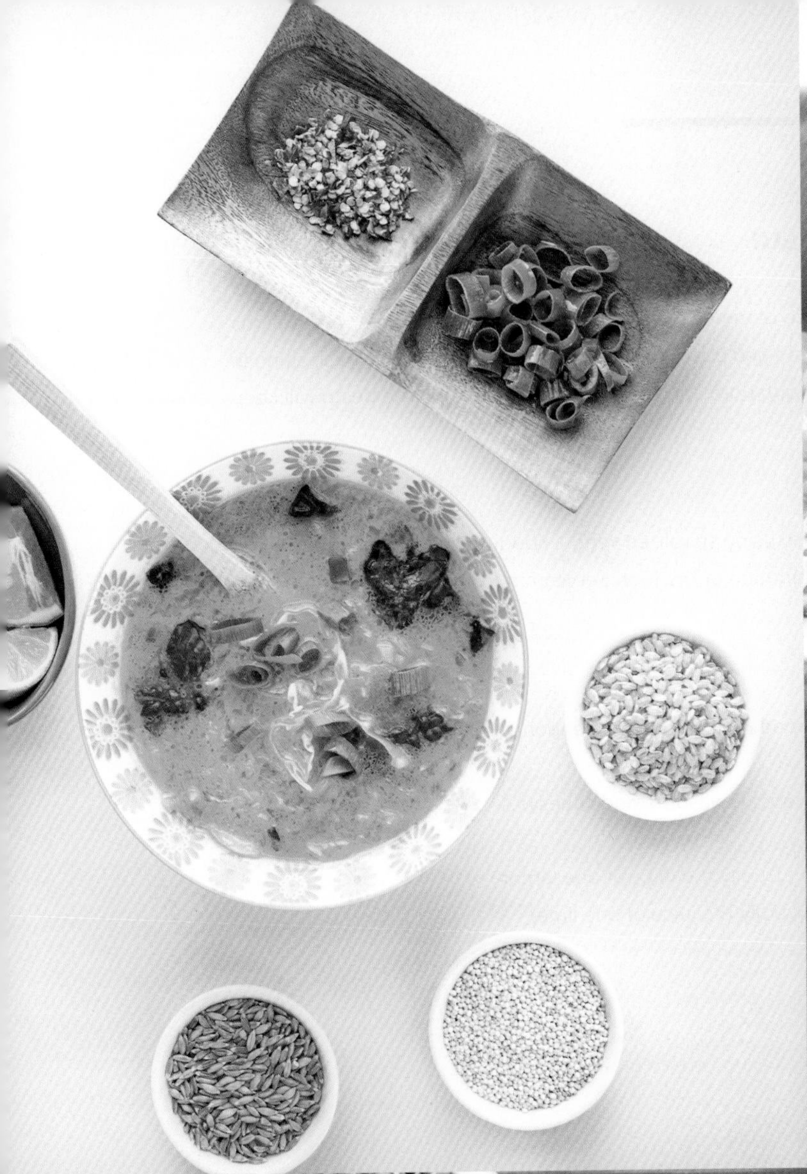

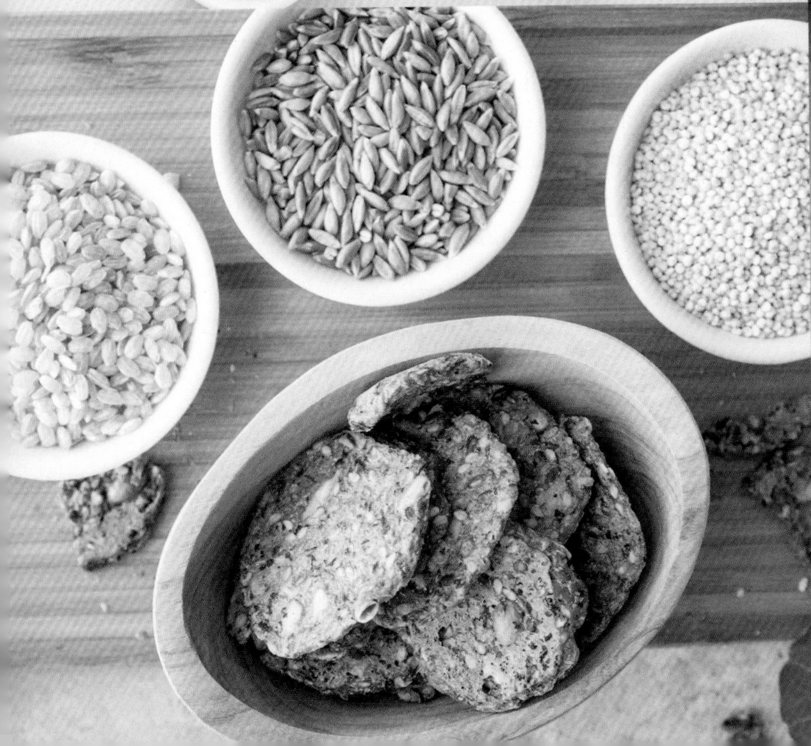

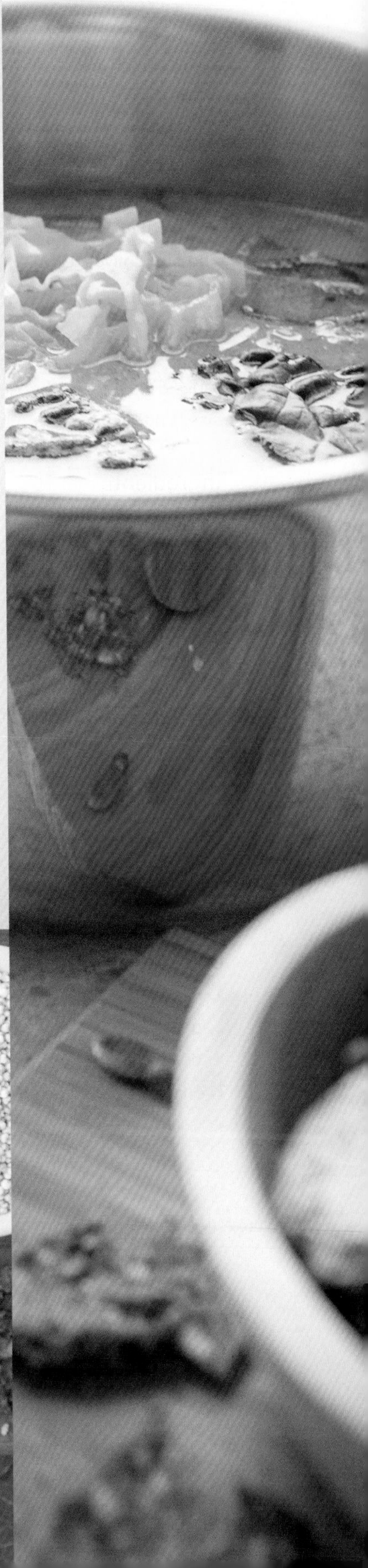

Walnut Basil Pesto

TOTAL PREP TIME **15 minutes**

Serve over pasta of choice alone or with anything your heart desires. A gorgeous combination is tossing pesto and pasta with grape or cherry tomatoes, fresh spinach and black olives. Garnish with basil sprigs and serve hot or cold! The pesto will keep for 5 days.

Tasty Tip

Make a completely raw dish using spiralized veggie noodles: zucchini, carrots, beets, sweet potato or any combination of the four. Serve immediately. Um, yum.

Ingredients

1 cup crushed walnuts

3 small cloves garlic- chopped (1 generous tablespoon)

¼ cup water

3 tablespoons nutritional yeast (awesome and cheesy)

2 tablespoons olive oil

2 tablespoons lemon juice (usually the juice of one lemon)

2 tablespoons lime juice (usually the juice of one lime)

1 tablespoon capers

1 tablespoon rice vinegar

½ teaspoon fine sea salt

4-5 cups fresh basil

More salt to taste

Some red pepper flakes (optional)

Directions

1. Place all the ingredients except basil in the bowl of a food processor fitted with a steel blade. Pulse a few times to combine, then with a rubber spatula, scrape down the sides of the bowl and continue to blend until smooth.
2. Add in basil and pulse to combine.

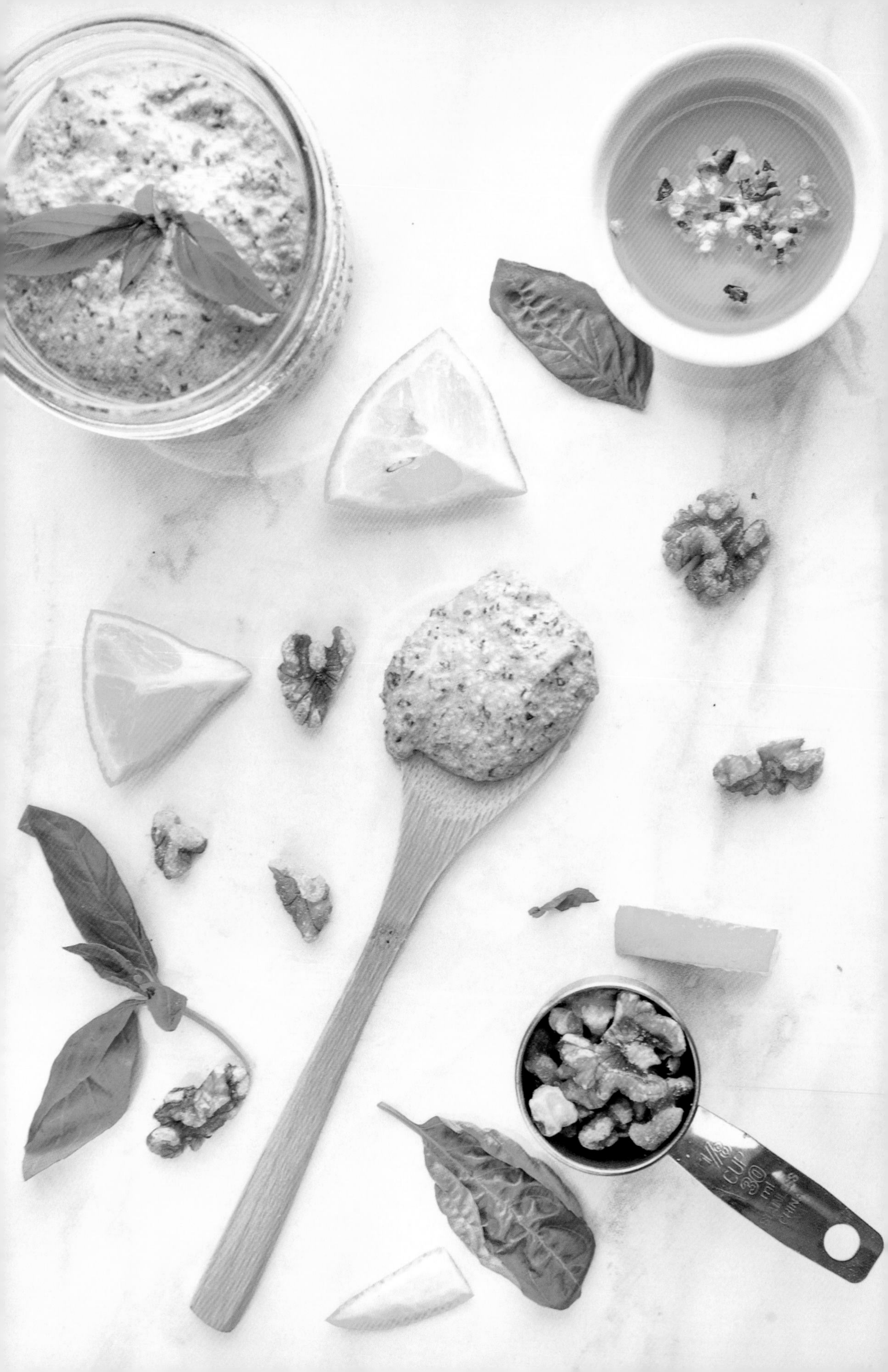
1/8
CUP
30

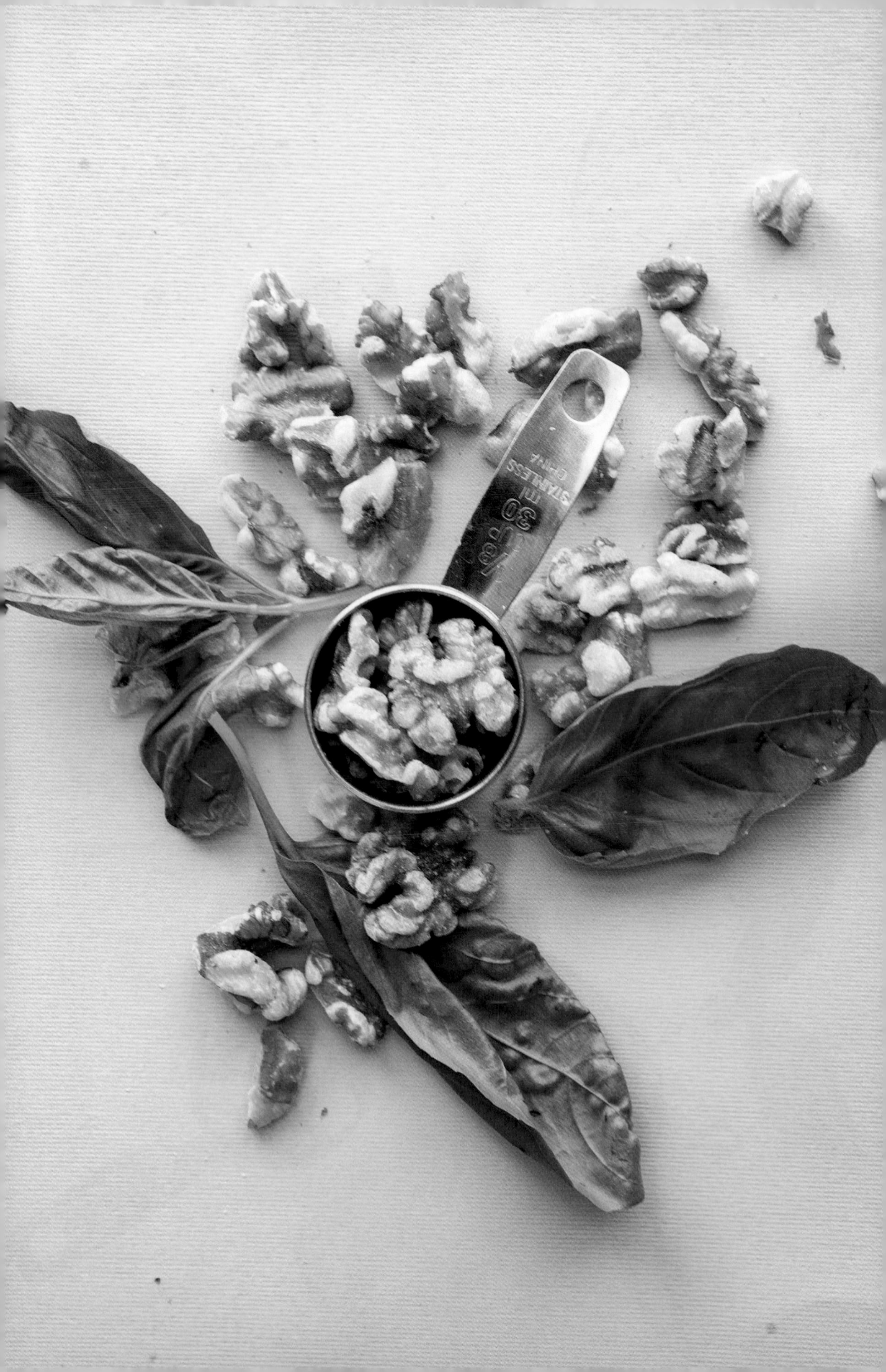
30 ml
STAINLESS
CHINA

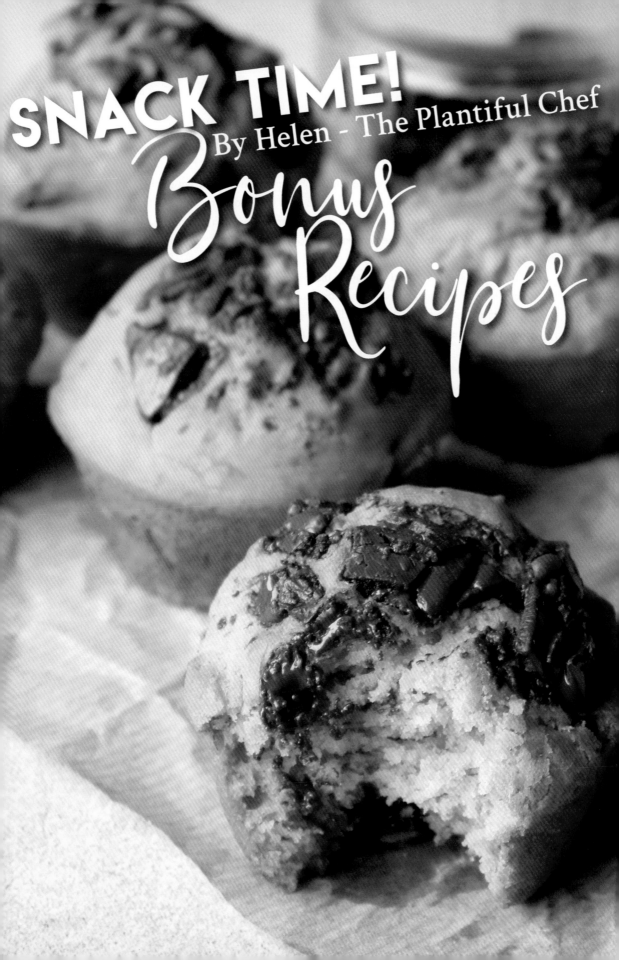

SNACK TIME!

By Helen - The Plantiful Chef

Bonus Recipes

Helen - The Plantiful Chef

Helen is the recipe developer and photographer and all around sweet toothed girl behind the blog, theplantifulchef.com. She is from Northeast England. She started her blog as a way of sharing her creations while embarking on a gluten-free / plant-based journey in order to ease her symptoms of Crohn's disease.

With an avid interest in food, and being trained as a chef before university over the years, Helen has had some amazing opportunities to work with some really high profile brands such as My Protein and Tesco. Her passion for health, wellness, and plant-based cuisine has also led to her getting paid to take pretty photos of food.

Helen has developed recipes to be featured in ebooks, including a blog version for the health brand Atkins. She recently became a published wellness writer with her article being published on healthline.com, the second leading health and website worldwide.

In her day job, she teaches adults and teenagers a wide variety of subjects. In the future, she aims to transition away from teaching and focus more on her career within the culinary industry. Helen's dream is to one day open up her own cafe and serve up some delicious plant-based food to her customers.

Helen absolutely loves hearing from her readers and anyone who comes across her work. Feel free to pop on over and say hello or drop her an Instagram direct message and tell her all about your experiences.

WWW.THEPLANTIFULCHEF.COM
ig: theplantifulchef | t: plantiful_chef

Vegan Banana Chocolate Muffins

Ingredients

2 small bananas mashed

¼ cup vegan butter

¼ cup coconut sugar

¼ cup dairy-free milk

2 teaspoons apple cider vinegar

1 teaspoon vanilla

1 cup flour = (buckwheat flour, almond flour, rice flour. If you want to make gluten-free muffins, you can also use gluten-free flour blends)

1 teaspoon baking powder

½ teaspoon baking soda

Vegan chocolate chunks / chips to desired amount

Directions

1. Preheat oven to 350F.
2. Mash the banana, butter, and sugar together in the bowl.
3. Once mashed, add in dairy-free milk, vanilla, and vinegar, and mix again.
4. Next, add in flour, baking powder, and baking soda.
5. Let mixture stand while you chop the chocolate.
6. Spoon micture into pre-greased muffin tins and sprinkle on chocolate and bake for around 20 minutes or until a toothpick comes out clean.

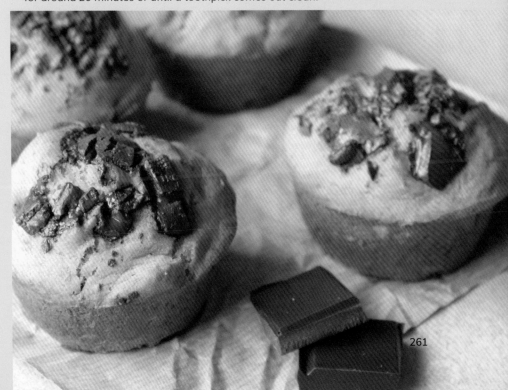

Gluten-free Crackers

PREP TIME 20 minutes

Ingredients

½ cup chickpea / gram flour

¼ cup buckwheat flour

¼ cup rice flour

½ teaspoon rosemary and thyme

¼ teaspoon garlic and onion powder

1 tablespoon olive oil

¼ cup water

More olive oil for brushing on the crackers

Directions

1. Mix all ingredients together until a solid dough forms. It might take a while but it will come together.
2. Roll out on a floured surface and cut into crackers.
3. Place cracker on a greaseproof paper on a baking tray and prick small holes with a fork in the cracker.
4. Bake at 400F for around 15 minutes.

Cheese And Chive Dip

PREP TIME 5 minutes

Ingredients

½ cup cashew soaked overnight

¼ cup of dairy-free creme fraiche or yogurt

2 tablespoons nutritional yeast

1 tablespoon apple cider vinegar

1 tablespoon lemon juice (usually the juice of half lemon)

1 tablespoon onion powder

10 chives chopped

Directions

1. Place everything in a blender apart from the chives and blend until smooth.
2. Stir in chives and place in the fridge for a few hours, works best if left overnight.
3. Garnish crackers with some cheese and chives on top. Enjoy!

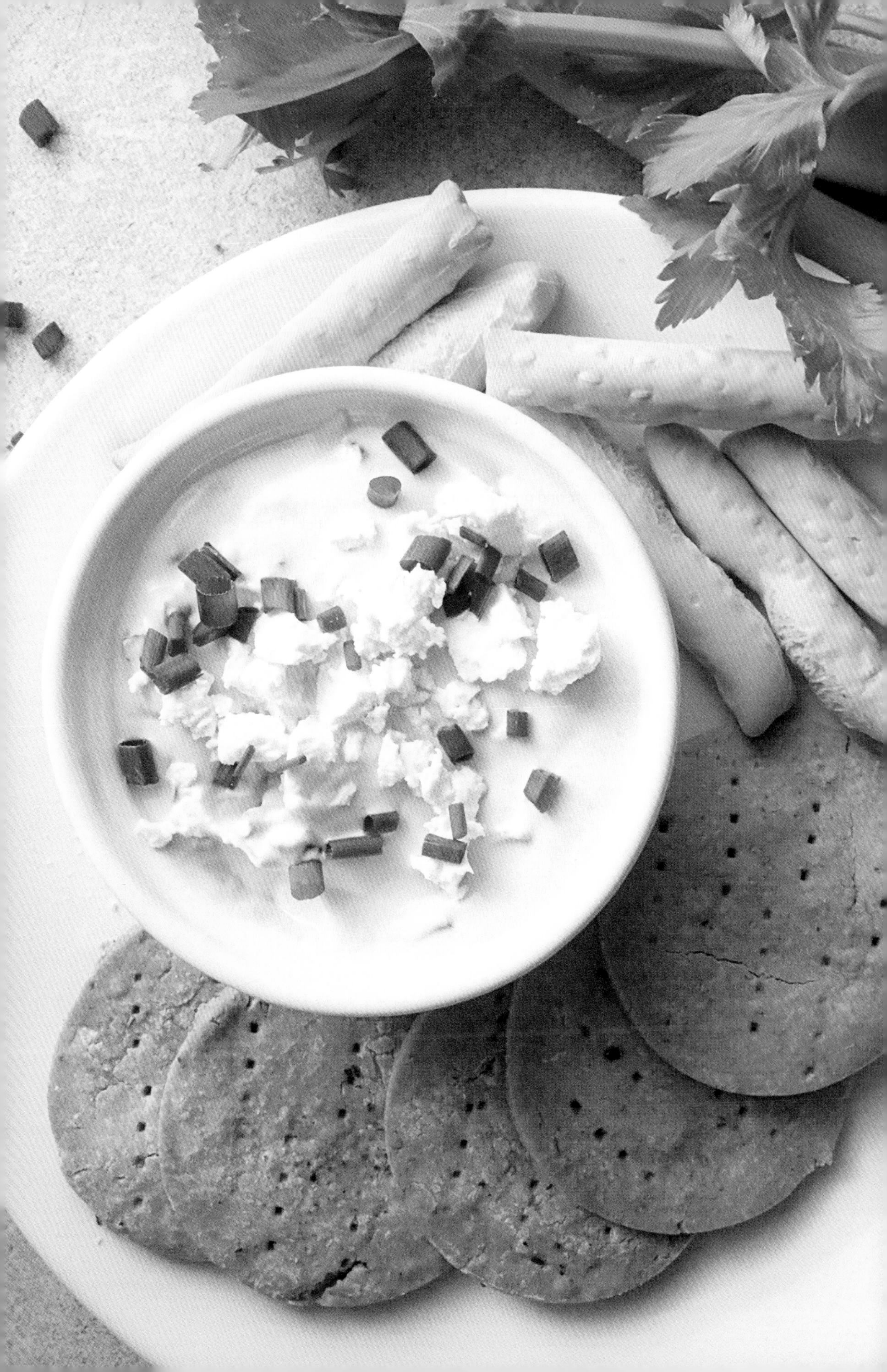

Coconut And Lime Energy Balls

PREP TIME **10 minutes**

Ingredients

1 cup cashew nuts

¼ cup desiccated coconut

¼ cup oats

2 tablespoons lime juice and zest (usually the zest and juice of one lime)

1 tablespoon agave syrup

More desiccated coconut to roll the energy balls in

Directions

1. Place cashews in blender and process until fine crumbs.

2. Then, place everything in a food processor and blend until sticky mixture forms.

3. Form mixture into 12 balls and roll in coconut.

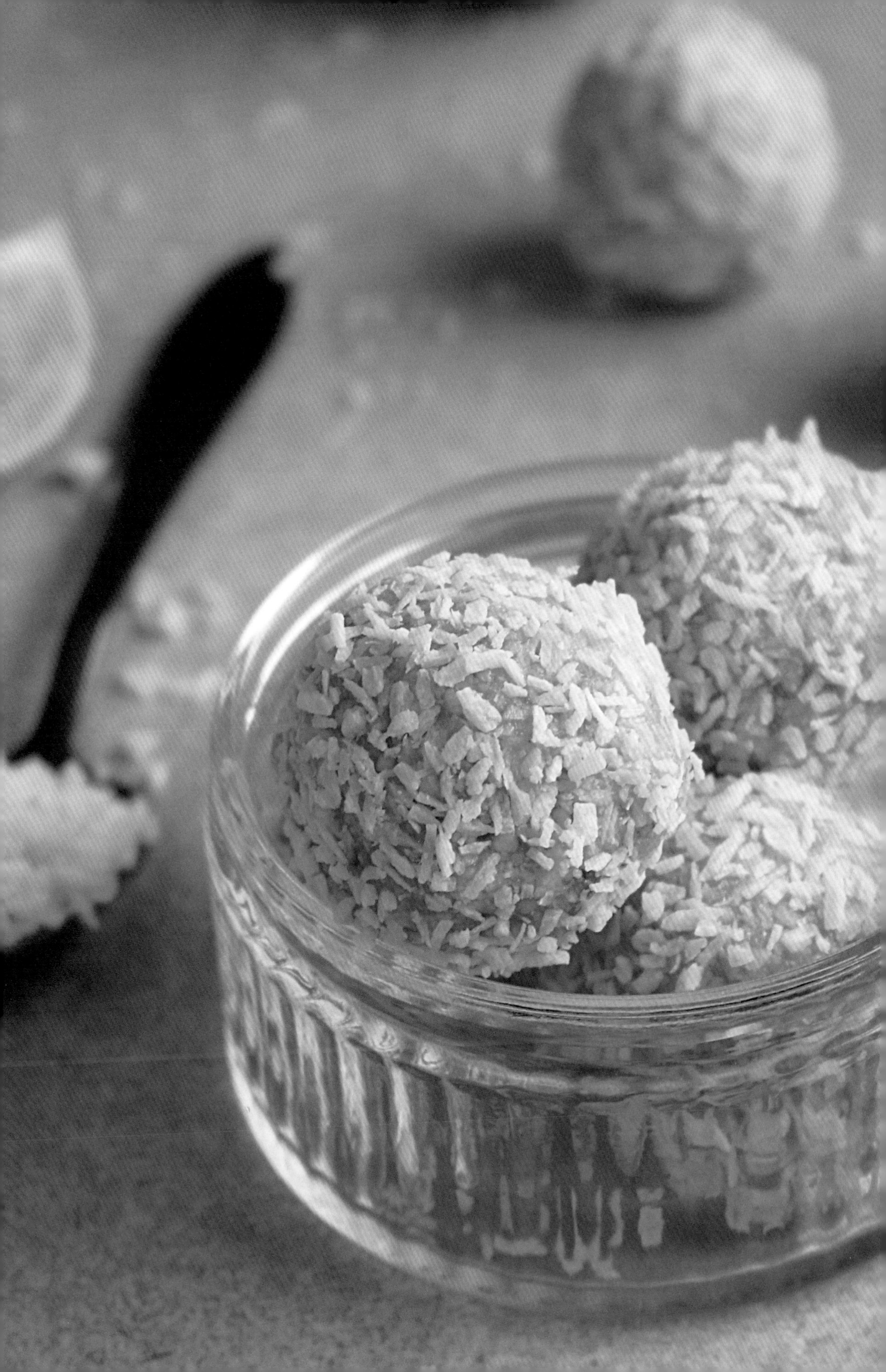

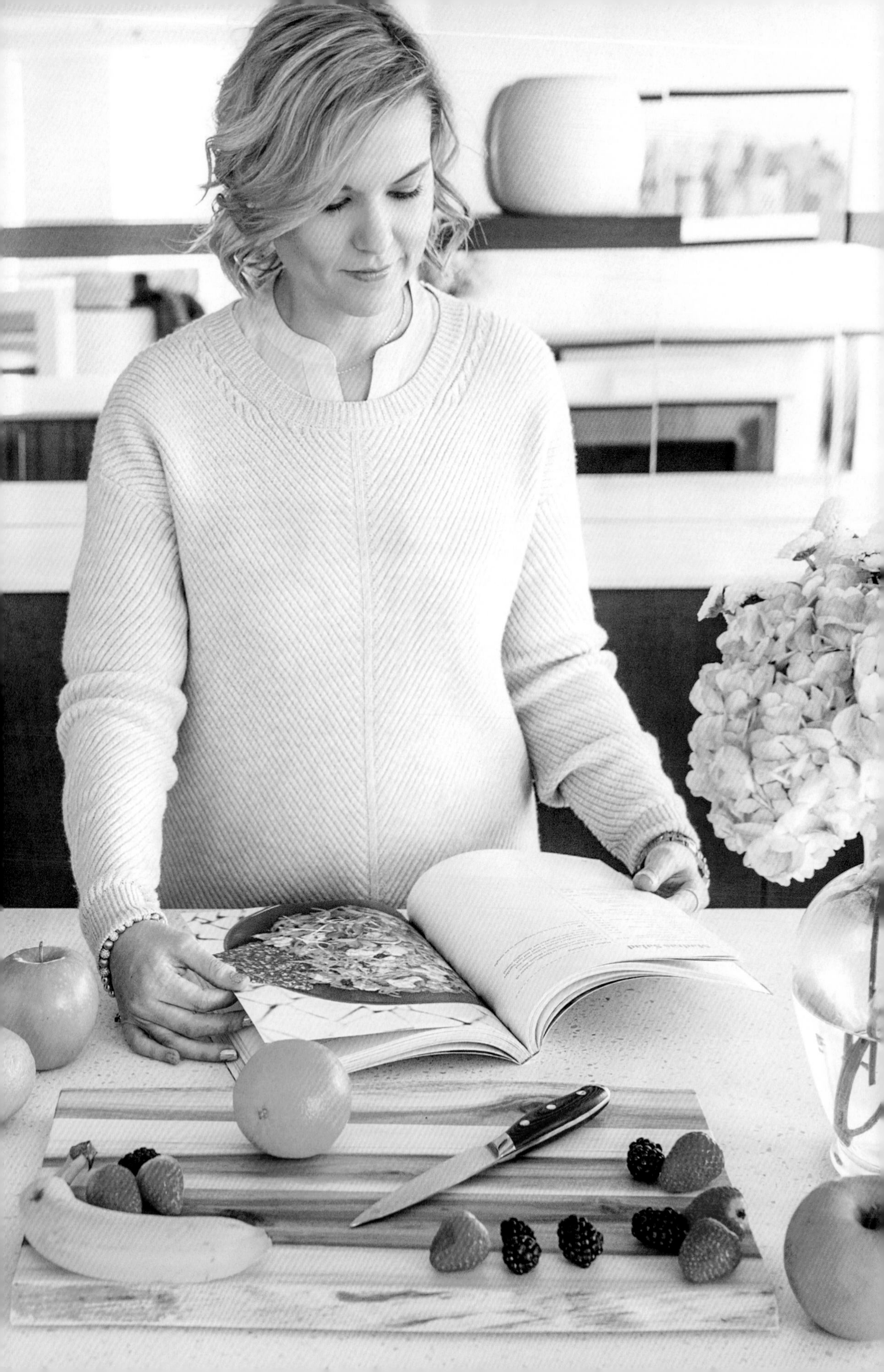

"BEEF" UP YOUR MEAL
THE UNEXPECTED MEAL-TOPPERS

by Ky-Lee Hanson

"BEEF" UP - AWESOME WAYS PLANT FOODS CAN ADD PROTEIN TO YOUR MEAL

Meat Alternatives / Replacements

We still want the meals we are accustomed to, without the cholesterol and animal cruelty. Many companies make great alternatives to beef, chicken, pork, or fish by using one or a combination of the following to achieve a palatable texture, then paired with the right seasonings:

- Tofu
- Soy protein
- Textured vegetable protein (TVP)
- Gluten protein (referred to as seitan below)
- Pea protein
- Legumes and beans: black bean, pinto, kidney, chickpea, peas, lentils
- Flours: chickpea, lentil, quinoa
- Mushrooms chopped, ground or steaked (sliced and marinated): Shiitake, king oyster mushroom, portobello to name a few varieties

To achieve the texture and flavor there are different processes you can look into or different premade products you can try.

Meal ideas: BBQ seitan "pork" | seitan (steak) | TVP beefless ground shepherd's pie | lentil no-meat loaf | tofu hot-dogs | veggie sausage | seitan steak | no-chick'n strips | a blend of these proteins with mushroom or corn make for a mean tasty veggie burger | vegan roast | TVP or lentil burger patty.

Remember bbq sauce, hickory smoke, and seasonings are what make meat palatable, we can achieve the same flavor with a different protein base.

TIP: Search the internet for meat alternatives followed by your country. You will see what is available to you via mail and find what brands are carried in stores near you. Call your local grocery store and health food store and ask what mock meats and alternatives they carry (milks, butters /spreads, cheese like foods, and faux meats). Some taste great, some are okay. You will need to find what suits you. Trying new foods is fun! Also search online or ask the retailers about health food and vegan festivals in your community so you can try samples.

Add Greens

For flavor, extra nutrients, and surprisingly high amounts of protein!
- Parsley
- Spinach
- Arugula

Meal ideas: on top of pizza or pasta | salad blends | in stir fry | pesto sauce | replace iceberg or romaine on a burger or sandwich

Seeds

- Source of protein and fiber while providing hearty flavor
- Chia powder or seeds
- Flaxseed or meal
- Sesame seeds
- Hemp hearts

Meal ideas: add to homemade bread | salad toppers | pudding or seed butters | add to shakes | thicken up sauces and make them hearty: chia in tomato sauce, sesame to make gomai

Protein Veggies

Broccoli

has more protein per calorie than beef [1]

Meal ideas: broccoli and mushroom (as a substitute for beef and mushroom) on rice | in pasta, fondue, pasta salad | on pizza | raw with hummus | roasted broccoli | broccoli slaw

Cauliflower

works too if you want a more subtle taste.

Meal ideas: cauliflower pizza crust | cauliflower mash | roasted cauliflower florets (chop, season, broil)

Brussel sprouts

The way to cook brussel sprouts is in a vegan butter alternative with a good dose of fresh lemon juice plus sea salt and pepper. I also like adding chili flakes!

Meal ideas: as cooked above: accompanying mashed potatoes and a vegan mock meat | drizzle balsamic glaze on top as a side dish with pizza or pasta | shaved leaves on top of salad, pasta, pizza | shaved into coleslaw

Dairy Alternatives

We provided a few recipes but here are some more ideas! Nuts blend into creme sauces simply with a nut milk, water, or vegetable stock in a regular blender. Garlic is key in flavor, lemon, salt, and pepper as well. Nutritional yeast has a cheesy flavor and usually also has Vitamin B12. Nut-based sauces are so creamy it is hard to tell that dairy is missing from the ingredients.

Common milk alternatives are almond, soy, cashew, and coconut milk. A favorite of mine is oat milk which is gluten free and naturally sweet! Hemp, pea, and rice are other alternatives.

Butter alternatives can be found in groceries stores as "vegan spreads." They are often a blend of oils with fortified vitamins. Avoid "natural flavor" and "artificial flavors" as there is no regulation on what these include. Other alternatives to butter are mashed avocados, cooking oils, butters / spreads made from pinenuts, cashew, peanut, almond, and coconut (refined equals no coconut taste), and blended white bean or chickpeas (hummus) for a creamy texture.

Meal ideas: vegan pistachio cream sauce on pasta | cashew spread | cashew & roasted eggplant dip | bean dip with cashew-sour-cream

Egg Alternatives

- Banana
- Flax egg replacement
- Apple sauce

Meal Ideas: The above can replace egg in bread | muffins | cookies
Breakfast: Avocado mash with black salt instead of scrambled eggs. Black salt is said to give the flavor of eggs while avocado provides protein and fat. It tastes delicious as a topping on toast, consider adding veggie sausage on the side.

GLOSSARY

A

Acupuncture: A treatment based on Chinese medicine. Thin needles are inserted into the skin at specific points on the body. This therapy is used to treat pain and various health problems and to reduce stress.

Adaptogens: A nontoxic substance and especially a plant extract that is held to increase the body's ability to resist the damaging effects of stress and promote or restore normal physiologivcal functioning.

Androgen: Any of a group of male sex hormones, including testosterone, that controls male characteristics such as beard growth.

Anthocyanins: Any of various soluble glycoside pigments producing blue to red coloring in flowers and plants.

Antimalarial: Serving to prevent, check, or cure malaria.

Antinuclear antibody (ANA) test: Antibodies that attack healthy proteins within the nucleus — the control center of your cells — are called antinuclear antibodies (ANA). When the body receives signals to attack itself, autoimmune diseases such as lupus, scleroderma, mixed connective tissue disease, autoimmune hepatitis, and others can occur. Symptoms vary by disease, but they may include rashes, swelling, arthritis, or fatigue. An ANA panel helps determine the level of ANA in your blood. You may have an autoimmune disorder if the level is high. However, conditions such as infections, cancer, and other medical problems can also result in a positive ANA test.

Ashwagandha: A preparation usually of the leaves or roots of an evergreen shrub (Withania somnifera) native to Africa, Asia, and southern Europe that is used in herbal medicine especially as a tonic, anti-inflammatory, and adaptogen.

Astragalus: (Astragalus membranaceus) has been used in Traditional Chinese Medicine (TCM) for thousands of years. Astragalus is called an adaptogen, meaning it helps protect the body against various stresses, including physical, mental, or emotional stress. Astragalus may help protect the body from diseases such as cancer and diabetes. Astragalus is used to protect and support the immune system, preventing colds and upper respiratory infections, lowering blood pressure, treating diabetes, and protecting the liver. Astragalus has antibacterial and anti-inflammatory properties.

B

Balanced translocation: The transfer of part of a chromosome to a different position especially on a nonhomologous chromosome; especially: The exchange of parts between nonhomologous chromosomes.

Barium enema: An examination of the large intestine using x-ray while injecting liquid into the rectum via a tube to gain a profile view of the intestine.

BHA: Probable carcinogen, produces liver damage, interferes with normal reproductive system development and thyroid hormone levels.

Biopsy: The removal of a small piece of tissue from the body for examination under a microscope.

Biotin: A colorless crystalline growth vitamin $C_{10}H_{16}N_2O_3S$ of the vitamin B complex found especially in yeast, liver, and egg yolk — called also vitamin H.

Boric Acid: Hormone disruptor.

C

C-reactive protein (CRP): A protein present in blood serum in various abnormal states (such as inflammation or neoplasia).

Calcium: A mineral that the body needs for many vital functions, including bone formation, regulation of heart rate and blood pressure, and muscle contraction.

Chaga mushroom: Chaga (Inonotus obliquus) is also known as Cinder Conk or Black Mass, which accurately describe ts appearance. The fruiting bodies of this mushroom contain polysaccharides, specifically a type called beta-glucans, which have been studied to support immune health and overall wellness, as well as normal, healthy cell growth and turnover. Chaga offers antioxidant support, and it is considered to be a tonic Mushroom to support overall wellness. It is used to promote healthy cell growth and turnover in the body, as well as gastrointestinal health.

Chelated: Means that a mineral is held in place by a larger molecule, such as an amino acid or other organic molecule. The mineral is held much like a claw would hold a small object. Chelation prevents a normally reactive mineral or ion like magnesium from interacting with other reactive substances. Chelation is common in naturally occurring chemicals but it can also be produced artificially for processing substances like magnesium when used in dietary supplements.

Coal tar hair dyes and other coal tar ingredients (including Aminophenol, Diaminobenzene, Phenylenediamine): Is a byproduct of coal processing and is a known human carcinogen.

Collagen: A fibrous protein that is the main component of connective tissue in the body.

Complete Blood Count (CBC): Is one of the most commonly ordered blood tests. The complete blood count is the calculation of the cellular (formed elements) of blood. A major portion of the complete blood count is the measure of the concentration of white blood cells, red blood cells, and platelets in the blood.

Comprehensive Metabolic Panel: (CMP) Is a blood test that gives doctors information about the body's fluid balance, levels of electrolytes like sodium and potassium, and how well the kidneys and liver are working.

Crohn's disease: A chronic disease that causes swelling of the digestive tract, pain, diarrhea.

D

Discoid Lupus Erythematosus: A rare form of lupus that causes a rash or scarring of skin.

Dyspepsia: Pain or discomfort in the upper abdomen; upset stomach or indigestion.

E

Eleutherococcus: This plant is found in North East China, Eastern Russia, Korea and Japan. It is used in Traditional Chinese Medicine to expel "Wind Dampness", to strengthen the sinews and bones, transform dampness and reduce swelling.

Endocrine disruptors: Chemicals that may interfere with the body's endocrine system and produce adverse developmental, reproductive, neurological, and immune effects in both humans and wildlife. A wide range of substances, both natural and manmade, are thought to cause endocrine disruption, including pharmaceuticals, dioxin and dioxin-like compounds, polychlorinated biphenyls, DDT and other pesticides, and plasticizers such as bisphenol A. Endocrine disruptors may be found in many everyday products– including plastic bottles, metal food cans, detergents, flame retardants, food, toys, cosmetics, and pesticides.

Endocrinologist: Are specially trained physicians who diagnose diseases related to the glands.

Endocrinology: A branch of medicine concerned with the structure, function, and disorders of the endocrine glands.

Endometrial Functions Test (EFT): Patients can now have their endometrium tested with the Endometrial Function Test® (EFT®). This patented test can optimize a patient's chances of having a successful pregnancy by using molecular markers to assess the endometrium's potential to support implantation and its ability to contribute to the nutrition of the developing embryo.

Erythrocyte sedimentation rate (ESR): An erythrocyte sedimentation rate (ESR) test is sometimes called a sedimentation rate test or sed rate test. This test doesn't diagnose one specific condition. Instead, it helps your doctor determine whether you're experiencing inflammation.

Estrogen: The main sex hormone in women.

F

Fluoroscopy: An x-ray procedure that makes it possible to see internal organs in motion.

Folate: Folate is a B-vitamin that is naturally present in many foods. A form of folate, known as folic acid, is used in dietary supplements and fortified foods. Our bodies need folate to make DNA and other genetic material. Folate is also needed for the body's cells to divide.

Folic acid: (also known as folate) is a B-vitamin found in many foods, including dark green leafy vegetables, fruits, nuts, beans, peas, dairy products, meat, eggs, and grains. It is required for the production of new cells and for proper synthesis of DNA. This vitamin is particularly important to a baby's health and development.

Formaldehyde releasers (Bronopol, DMDM hydantoin, Diazolidinyl urea, Imidzaolidinyl urea, and Quaternium-15): Cosmetics preservatives that slowly form formaldehyde to kill bacteria growing in products. Formaldehyde is a known human carcinogen. The preservatives and the formaldehyde they generate can trigger allergic
skin reactions.

Formaldehyde: Known carcinogen; also an asthmagen, neurotoxicant, and developmental toxicant.

Fragrance: This one term can legally hide hundreds of chemicals, including phthalates, which are known endocrine disruptors. Foregoing fragrance does not mean having to live stinky. Many companies are now offering safe personal-care alternatives that are naturally scented with pure essential oils.

G

Ginseng: There are two types of Ginseng - American Ginseng and Asian Ginseng. A member of the araliaceae (Ivy) family, and in the same genus as Asian (or Korean) Ginseng (Panax ginseng), these two plants are closely related in use, yet American Ginseng has a reputation of being much less stimulating and more "cooling". Ginseng is used to tonify digestion, and to support normal energy.

H

Hemoglobin: A red protein responsible for transporting oxygen in the blood of vertebrates. Its molecule comprises four subunits, each containing an iron atom bound to a heme group.

Hirschsprung's disease: A congenital condition where a portion of the large intestine has a complete absence of nerves and motility.

Holy Basil: Also an adaptogen, Holy Basil has been used to support a healthy response to stress, maintain blood sugar levels within a normal range, has anti-inflammatoryproperties, promote longevity, nourish mind & elevate spirit.

Homeostasis: The tendency of the body to seek and maintain a condition of balance or equilibrium within its internal environment, even when faced with external changes.

Hot flashes: A sudden, intense, hot feeling in the face or upper part of the body, along with rapid heartbeat, sweating, and flushing. A symptom of menopause.

Hypothalamus: A small area in the brain that produces hormones that control body temperature, hunger, moods, the stress response, and other key functions.

I

Inositol: Inositol, sometimes called vitamin B8, is one of the B complex vitamins that the body needs in small amounts daily to stay healthy. However it is not officially recognised as a vitamin as it can be synthesized in the body from glucose, by intestinal bacteria. The most common natural form of it is myo-inositol.

Integrative Medicine: Integrative medicine is healing-oriented medicine that takes account of the whole person (body, mind, and spirit), including all aspects of lifestyle. It emphasizes the therapeutic relationship and makes use of all appropriate therapies, both conventional and alternative.

Iridology: Iridology (pronounced eye-ri-dology) is the art and science of analyzing the color and structure of the iris to determine tissue integrity throughout the body. Iridology is a form of analysis that is non-invasive to the body, requiring no x-raying or use of any other invasive techniques to complete the analysis.

Isothiocyanates: A family of organic compounds found in tangy herbs such as horseradish, mustard, and onions. They have several patented applications including use as a pesticide, and their presence in the diet is thought to help prevent cancer in humans.

IVF: In Vitro Fertilization is an assisted reproductive technology (ART) commonly referred to as IVF. IVF is the process of fertilization by extracting eggs, retrieving a sperm sample, manually combining an egg and sperm in a laboratory dish. The embryo(s) is then transferred to the uterus.

L

Loop Electrosurgical Excision Procedure (LEEP): Uses an electric current passed through a loop of thin wire to remove abnormal tissue from the cervix. The loop of wire acts like a scalpel to remove the tissue. LEEP may also be called large loop excision of the transformation zone (LLETZ) or a loop excision.

Lutein: (pronounced loo-teen), like zeaxanthin is an antioxidant that is located in the eye. Green leafy vegetables, as well as other foods such as eggs, contain these important nutrients. Many studies have shown that lutein and zeaxanthin reduce the risk of chronic eye diseases, including AMD and cataracts.

Lycopene: Is a naturally occurring chemical that gives fruits and vegetables a red color. It is one of a number of pigments called carotenoids. Lycopene is found in watermelons, pink grapefruits, apricots, and pink guavas. It is found in particularly high amounts in tomatoes and tomato products. It protects the cells from damage, prevents heart disease, "hardening of the arteries" (atherosclerosis); and cancer of the prostate, breast, lung, bladder, ovaries, colon, and pancreas. Lycopene is also used for treating human papilloma virus (HPV) infection, which is a major cause of uterine cancer. Some people also use lycopene for cataracts and asthma.

Magnesium: Is one of the many minerals the body needs for normal muscles, nerves, and bones. It also helps keep a steady heart rhythm, a healthy immune system, normal blood sugar levels and blood pressure, and is involved in making energy and protein for the body. Magnesium is found in some foods, including green vegetables, beans and peas, nuts and seeds, and whole grainst.

Manganese: Is a naturally occurring mineral in our bodies in very small amounts. It is an actual component of manganese superoxide dismutase enzyme. It is a powerful antioxidant that seeks out the free radicals in the human body and neutralizes these damaging particles, thereby preventing many of the potential dangers they cause. The health benefits of manganese include healthy bones and better metabolism. It also acts as a coenzyme to assist metabolic activities in the human body. Apart from these, there are other health benefits of manganese including the formation of connective tissues, absorption of calcium, proper functioning of the thyroid gland and sex hormones, regulation of blood sugar level, and proper metabolism of fats and carbohydrates.

Methylisothiazolinone, methylchloroisothiazolinone and benzisothiazolinone: Preservatives, commonly used together in personal care products, are among the most common irritants, sensitizers, and causes of contact allergy. Lab studies on mammalian brain cells suggest that methylisothiazolinone may be neurotoxic.

Microbiota: Is an "ecological community of commensal, symbiotic and pathogenic microorganisms" found in and on all multicellular organisms studied to date from plants to animals. A microbiota includes bacteria, archaea, protists, fungi and viruses.

Monounsaturated fats: From a chemical standpoint, are simply fat molecules that have one unsaturated carbon bond in the molecule, this is also called a double bond. Oils that contain monounsaturated fats are typically liquid at room temperature but start to turn solid when chilled. Olive oil is an example of a type of oil that contains monounsaturated fats.

Naturopath: Naturopathic physicians combine the wisdom of nature with the rigors of modern science. Steeped in traditional healing methods, principles and practices, naturopathic medicine focuses on holistic, proactive prevention and comprehensive diagnosis and treatment.

Niacin: Is also known as vitamin B and has 2 other forms, niacinamide (nicotinamide) and inositol hexanicotinate, which have different effects from niacin. All B vitamins help the body convert food (carbohydrates) into fuel (glucose), which the body uses to produce energy. These B vitamins, often referred to as B-complex vitamins, also help the body use fats and protein. B-complex vitamins are needed for a healthy liver, healthy skin, hair, and eyes, and to help the nervous system function properly. Niacin also helps the body make various sex and stress-related hormones in the adrenal glands and other parts of the body. Niacin helps improve circulation, and it has been shown to suppress inflammation.

O

Ovarian cysts: Are fluid-filled sacs or pockets in an ovary or on its surface. Women have two ovaries — each about the size and shape of an almond — on each side of the uterus. Eggs (ova), which develop and mature in the ovaries, are released in monthly cycles during the childbearing years.

Oxybenzone: Is a sunscreen ingredient associated with photoallergic reactions. This chemical absorbs through the skin in significant amounts. It contaminates the bodies of 97% of Americans according to research by the Centers for Disease Control and Prevention.

P

Pantothenic acid: Vitamin B5, also called pantothenic acid, is one of 8 B vitamins. In addition to playing a role in the breakdown of fats and carbohydrates for energy, vitamin B5 is critical to the manufacture of red blood cells, as well as sex and stress-related hormones produced in the adrenal glands, small glands that sit atop the kidneys. Vitamin B5 is also important in maintaining a healthy digestive tract, and it helps the body use other vitamins, particularly B2 (also called riboflavin). It is sometimes called the "anti-stress" vitamin, but there is no concrete evidence whether it helps the body withstand stress. Your body needs pantothenic acid to synthesize cholesterol. Vitamin B5 deficiency is rare, but may include symptoms such as fatigue, insomnia, depression, irritability, vomiting, stomach pains, burning feet, and upper respiratory infections.

Parabens (specifically Propyl-, Isopropyl-, Butyl-, and Isobutyl): Are estrogen-mimicking preservatives used widely in cosmetics. They may disrupt the endocrine system and cause reproductive and developmental disorders.

Polycystic Ovarian Syndrome (PCOS): Is a hormonal disorder common among women of reproductive age. Women with PCOS may have infrequent or prolonged menstrual periods or excess male hormone (androgen) levels. The ovaries may develop numerous small collections of fluid (follicles) and fail to regularly release eggs.

PEGs/Ceteareth/Polyethylene compounds: These synthetic chemicals are frequently contaminated with 1,4-dioxane, which the U.S. government considers a probable human carcinogen and which readily penetrates the skin.

Peristalsis: Is a series of wave-like muscle contractions that moves food to different processing stations in the digestive tract. The process of peristalsis begins in the esophagus when a bolus of food is swallowed.

Phenolic: Any of the class of thermosetting resins formed by the condensation of phenol, or of a phenol derivative, with an aldehyde, especially formaldehyde: used chiefly in the manufacture of paints and plastics and as adhesives for sandpaper and plywood.

Phosphorus: Is a mineral found in your bones. Along with calcium, phosphorus is needed to build strong healthy bones, as well as, keeping other parts of your body healthy.

Phthalates: Are a group of chemicals used in plastics to soften and increase flexibility. Phthalates affect reproductive organs and hormones, especially in prepubescent males. Some have been linked to breast and other cancers, allergies, obesity, thyroid, and other hormonal disruption. They may damage the male reproductive system. It is not required to be labeled as it can legally be hidden under the ingredient "fragrance," "parfum," etc.

Phytochemicals: Are non-nutritive plant chemicals that have protective or disease preventive properties. They are non-essential nutrients, meaning that they are not required by the human body for sustaining life. It is well-known that plants produce these chemicals to protect themselves but recent research demonstrate that they can also protect humans against diseases. There are more than thousand known phytochemicals. Some of the well-known phytochemicals are lycopene in tomatoes, isoflavones in soy and flavonoids in fruits.

Phytosterols: (referred to as plant sterol and stanol esters) are a group of naturally occurring compounds found in plant cell membranes. Because phytosterols are structurally similar to the body's cholesterol, when they are consumed they compete with cholesterol for absorption in the digestive system. As a result, cholesterol absorption is blocked, and blood cholesterol levels reduced.

Pituitary gland: Is a tiny organ, the size of a pea, found at the base of the brain. As the "master gland" of the body, it produces many hormones that travel throughout the body, directing certain processes or stimulating other glands to produce other hormones. The pituitary gland produces prolactin, which acts on the breasts to induce milk production. The pituitary gland also secretes hormones that act on the adrenal glands, thyroid gland, ovaries and testes, which in turn produce other hormones. Through secretion of its hormones, the pituitary gland controls metabolism, growth, sexual maturation, reproduction, blood pressure and many other vital physical functions and processes.

Pleurisy: Inflammation of the lining of the lung and inner chest wall.

Premenstrual Dysphoric Disorder (PMDD): Is a condition in which a woman has severe depression symptoms, irritability, and tension before menstruation. The symptoms of PMDD are more severe than those seen with premenstrual syndrome (PMS).

Premenstrual Symptoms (PMS): Refers to a wide range of physical or emotional symptoms that most often occur about 5 to 11 days before a woman starts her monthly menstrual cycle. In most cases, the symptoms stop when, or shortly after, her period begins.

Postpartum depression (PPD): Also called postnatal depression, is a type of mood disorder associated with childbirth, which can affect both sexes. Symptoms may include extreme sadness, low energy, anxiety, crying episodes, irritability, and changes in sleeping or eating patterns.

Potassium: Is a mineral that is found in the foods you eat. It is also an electrolyte. Electrolytes conducts electrical impulses throughout the body. They assist in a range of essential body functions such as regulating and maintaining blood pressure, normal water balance, muscle contractions, nerve impulses, digestion, heart rhythm, pH balance (acidity and alkalinity).

Phosphorus: Is a mineral found in your bones. Along with calcium, phosphorus is needed to build strong healthy bones, as well as, keeping other parts of your body healthy.

Preimplantation Genetic Diagnosis (PGD): Is a procedure used prior to implantation to help identify genetic defects within embryos. This serves to prevent certain genetic diseases or disorders from being passed on to the child. The embryos used in PGD are usually created during the process of in vitro fertilization (IVF).

Proanthocyanins (PAs): Also known as condensed tannins, are very powerful antioxidants that remove harmful free oxygen radicals from cells. Studies indicate that antioxidant power of proanthocyanidins is 20 times higher than that of vitamin C and 50 times higher than vitamin E.

Progesterone: Is one of the progesterone steroid hormones. It is secreted by the corpus luteum, a temporary endocrine gland that the female body produces after ovulation during the second half of the menstrual cycle.

Post Traumatic Stress Disorder (PTSD): Is a disorder that develops in some people who have experienced a shocking, scary, or dangerous event. Fear triggers many split-second changes in the body to help defend against danger or to avoid it. This "fight-or-flight" response is a typical reaction meant to protect a person from harm. Nearly everyone will experience a range of reactions after trauma, yet most people recover from initial symptoms naturally. Those who continue to experience problems may be diagnosed with PTSD. People who have PTSD may feel stressed or frightened even when they are not in danger.

R

Reishi mushroom (Ganoderma lucidum): An edible type of medicinal fungus that has been used for various healing abilities for thousands of years, is a true "superfood." Also known as Ling Zhi in Chinese, these mushrooms are strongly anti-inflammatory and tied to longevity, better immune function and mental clarity — perhaps that's why they've adopted the nickname "king of mushrooms."

R.E.M sleep: A kind of sleep that occurs at intervals during the night and is characterized by rapid eye movements, more dreaming and bodily movement, and faster pulse and breathing.

Resorcinol: Is a common ingredient in hair color and bleaching products. It is a skin irritant, and is toxic to the immune system and a frequent cause of hair dye allergy. In animal studies, resorcinol can disrupt normal thyroid function.

Rhodiola rosea: Is the fragrant root of an herb believed to have adaptogenic properties. That is, it helps the body adapt to internal and external stressors. Also called golden root, arctic root, and roseroot, Rhodiola rosea has been used medicinally for centuries. The extract commonly serves as an enhancement supplement, increasing performance and endurance. It's also thought to decrease fatigue, stress, and depression. As well, it's been used to treat infections, nervous system disorders, and even cancer.

Riboflavin: Also known as vitamin B2, Riboflavin is one of eight B vitamins.

S

Selenium: Is a trace mineral found naturally in the soil that also appears in certain high-selenium foods, and there are even small amounts in water. It is an extremely vital mineral for the human body as it increases immunity, takes part in antioxidant activity that defends against free radical damage and inflammation, and plays a key role in maintaining a healthy metabolism. According to studies, consuming plenty of naturally occurring selenium has positive antiviral effects, is essential for successful male and female fertility and reproduction, and also reduces the risk of cancer, autoimmune and thyroid diseases.

Sodium borate: Hormone disruptor.

Systemic lupus erythematosus (SLE): Is an autoimmune disease. In this disease, the body's immune system mistakenly attacks healthy tissue. It can affect the skin, joints, kidneys, brain, and other organs.

T

Thiamin (vitamin B1): Helps the body's cells change carbohydrates into energy. The main role of carbohydrates is to provide energy for the body, especially the brain and nervous system. Thiamin also plays a role in muscle contraction and conduction of nerve signals, and is essential for the metabolism of pyruvate. Thiamin can be found in enriched, fortified, and whole grain products such as bread, cereals, rice, pasta, and flour, wheat germ, beef steak and pork, trout and bluefin tuna, egg, legumes and peas, nuts and seeds.

Toluene: Found in paint thinner and nail polish. May impair fetal development. Has been associated with toxicity to the immune system. Some evidence suggests a link to malignant lymphoma.

Triclosan & Triclocarban: Antimicrobial agents - typically the active ingredient in antibacterial soaps, lotions and other products. These two ingredients are linked to endocrine disruption and reproductive issues, and overuse may promote the development of bacterial resistance.

Tui Na: The term tui na (pronounced "twee naw"), which literally means "pinch and pull," refers to a wide range of Traditional Chinese Medicine (TCM) therapeutic massage and bodywork. As such, practitioners use it for many of the same reasons and according to the same principles as acupuncture. Like acupuncture, TCM uses tui na to harmonize yin and yang in the body by manipulating the Qi in the acupuncture channels. Tui na includes what is popularly known as "acupressure," where practitioners use finger pressure instead of needles to stimulate the acupuncture points.

U

Unbalanced translocation: A translocation means that there is an unusual arrangement of the chromosomes.

Urethropscopy with dilation: An examination of the urethra using a scope, a ureteral balloon is used to dilate and stretch the urethra to prevent urinary tract infections.

Urethroscopy: An examination of the urethra using a scope.

Urinalysis: A urinalysis is a test of your urine and is used to detect and manage a wide range of disorders, such as urinary tract infections, kidney disease and diabetes.

Urinary tract infection: An infection in any part of the urinary tract causing, burning, urgency, pain, bloody urine, and sometimes lower back pain.

Vitamin A compounds (retinyl palmitate, retinyl acetate, retinol): When applied topically, can increase skin irritation and accelerate skin cancer growth.

Yellow Maca: Contains nearly all essential amino acids and free fatty acids, significant levels of vitamins A, B1, B2, B3, and C, minerals, iron, magnesium, zinc and calcium, a high concentration of bioavailable protein and nutrients unique to Maca called macaenes and macamides. It is also an adaptogen, or a rare form of plants that is thought to raise the overall life force energy of those who consume it. Yellow Maca boosts energy, promotes fertility and hormonal balance, increases mental focus, and aids with maintaining overall health and well-being.

Z

Zeaxanthin: (pronounced zee-uh-zan-thin): Are antioxidants that are located in the eye. Green leafy vegetables, as well as other foods such as eggs, contain these important nutrients. Studies have shown that zeaxanthin reduce the risk of chronic eye diseases: AMD, cataracts.

Citations

Introduction

1. Publishing, H. H. (n.d.). Red meat: Avoid the processed stuff. Retrieved from https://www.health.harvard.edu/family-health-guide/updates/red-meat-avoid-the-processed-stuff

2. McGruther, J. (n.d.). Nutrient Showdown: Best Sources of Vitamins & Minerals [Web log post]. Retrieved from http://nourishedkitchen.com/best-sources-vitamins-minerals/
Additional Resources

3. Melone, L. (2015, November 19). 10 Reasons To Stop Eating Red Meat. Retrieved from https://www.prevention.com/food/healthy-eating-tips/10-reasons-to-stop-eating-red-meat/slide/4

4. McClees, H. (2015, March 23). Nutrients Found in Meat That You Can Get From Plants Instead. Retrieved http://www.onegreenplanet.org/natural-health/nutrients-found-in-meat-you-can-get-from-plants-instead/

5. Plant-Based Protein VS. Protein From Meat: Which One Is Better For Your Body? (2016, October 06). Retrieved from http://www.collective-evolution.com/2016/09/27/plant-based-protein-vs-protein-from-meat-which-one-is-better-for-your-body-dont-publish-waiting-for-picture/

Chapter 1 - Finding Balance In Today's World - by Rebecca Hall

1. Ronald J. Garan Jr. (2018, April 09). Retrieved from https://en.wikipedia.org/wiki/Ronald_J._Garan_Jr.

2. Current World Population. (n.d.). Retrieved from http://www.worldometers.info/world-population/

3. How much do oceans add to world's oxygen? (n.d.). Retrieved from http://earthsky.org/earth/how-much-do-oceans-add-to-worlds-oxygen

4. Brighty, G. C., Jones, D., & Ruxton, J. (n.d.). High-Level Science Review for 'A Plastic Oceans' Film [Review]. Retrieved from https://plasticoceans.org/wp-content/uploads/2017/01/Plastic-Oceans-High-Level-Science-Summary-Version-4.pdf

5. Arizona State University (2010, March 20). Impact of plastics on human health and ecosystems. Retrieved from https://www.news-medical.net/news/20100320/Impact-of-plastics-on-human-health-and-ecosystems.aspx

6. Endocrine system. (2018, April 09). Retrieved from https://en.wikipedia.org/wiki/Endocrine_system

7. Plant-based diets could save millions of lives and dramatically cut greenhouse gas emissions. (2016, March 21). Retrieved from https://www.oxfordmartin.ox.ac.uk/news/201603_Plant_based_diets

8. Shilhavy, B. (n.d.). ALERT: Certified Organic Food Grown in U.S. Found Contaminated with Glyphosate Herbicide. Retrieved from http://healthimpactnews.com/2014/alert-certified-organic-food-grown-in-u-s-found-contaminated-with-glyphosate-herbicide/

9. Beville, R. (2016, July 13). HOW PERVASIVE ARE GMOS IN ANIMAL FEED? Retrieved from http://www.gmoinside.org/gmos-in-animal-feed/

10. World's Number 1 Herbicide Discovered in U.S. Mothers' Breast Milk. (2014, April 27). Retrieved from https://sustainablepulse.com/2014/04/06/worlds-number-1-herbicide-discovered-u-s-mothers-breast-milk/#.WsyKppPwbOT

11. Jandhyala, S. M., Talukdar, R., Subramanyam, C., Vuyyuru, H., Sasikala, M., & Reddy, D. N. (2015, August 07). Role of the normal gut microbiota. World Journal of Gastroenterology : WJG, 21(29), 8787–8803. http://doi.org/10.3748/wjg.v21.i29.8787

12. Samsel, A., & Seneff, S. (2013, April 18). Glyphosate's Suppression of Cytochrome P450 Enzymes and Amino Acid Biosynthesis by the Gut Microbiome: Pathways to Modern Diseases†. Retrieved from http://www.mdpi.com/1099-4300/15/4/1416

13. Chow, L. (2017, October 25). Human Exposure to Glyphosate Has Skyrocketed 500% Since Introduction of GMO Crops. Retrieved from https://www.ecowatch.com/glyphosate-exposure-humans-2501317778.html

14. Schippa, S., & Pia Conte, M. (2014, December 11). Dysbiotic Events in Gut Microbiota: Impact on Human Health. Retrieved from http://www.mdpi.com/2072-6643/6/12/5786

15. Alternative Medicine. (n.d.). Retrieved from http://www.umm.edu/health/medical/altmed/condition/intestinal-parasites

16. Reece, M., PhD. (n.d.). What is pH Balance? Retrieved from https://www.medicalsciencenavigator.com/what-is-ph-balance/

17. Felts, L., CN. (2015, January 23). Acid to Alkaline: The 80 Best Foods for Balancing Your pH Levels. Retrieved from http://thechalkboardmag.com/acid-to-alkaline-the-best-foods-for-boosting-your-ph-levels

18. Spirulina (dietary supplement). (2018, April 09). Retrieved from https://en.wikipedia.org/wiki/Spirulina_(dietary_supplement)

19. Serotonin. (2018, April 09). Retrieved April 10, 2018, from https://en.wikipedia.org/wiki/Serotonin

20. Glover, Vivette et al. (2002, December). Benefits of infant massage for mothers with postnatal depression. Seminars in Neonatology , Volume 7 , Issue 6 , 495 - 500. Retrieved from http://www.sfnmjournal.com/article/S1084-2756(02)90154-5/pdf

21. Cortisol. (2018, April 09). Retrieved April 10, 2018, from https://en.wikipedia.org/wiki/Cortisol

22. Adaptogenic Plants. (n.d.). Retrieved from http://www.adaptogens.org/original/adaptogenic plants.htm

23. 21 Surprising Benefits Of Aloe Vera. (n.d.). Retrieved from https://www.organicfacts.net/health-benefits/herbs-and-spices/health-benefits-of-aloe-vera.html

24. Monaco, E. (n.d.). 35 Amazing Wheatgrass Benefits for Health, Hair and Beauty (Backed by Science!). Retrieved from http://www.organicauthority.com/benefits-of-wheatgrass.html

25. Chelation. (2018, April 09). Retrieved from https://en.wikipedia.org/wiki/Chelation

26. Pandey, K. B., & Rizvi, S. I. (2009). Plant polyphenols as dietary antioxidants in human health and disease. Oxidative Medicine and Cellular Longevity, 2(5), 270–278.

27. Melatonin. (2018, April 09). Retrieved from https://en.wikipedia.org/wiki/Melatonin

28. Bell, P. G., Gaze, D. C., Davison, G. W., George, T. W., Scotter, M. J., & Howatson, G. (2014). Montmorency tart cherry (Prunus cerasus L.) concentrate lowers uric acid, independent of plasma cyanidin-3-O-glucosiderutinoside. Journal Of Functional Foods,11, 82-90. doi:https://doi.org/10.1016/j.jff.2014.09.004

29. Seymour E, Warber S, Kirakosyan A, et al. Anthocyanin pharmacokinetics and dose-dependent plasma antioxidant pharmacodynamics following whole tart cherry intake in healthy humans. Journal of Functional Foods. 2014.

Chapter 2 - A Toxic Agenda - by Meghan Rose

1. Price, J. H., Khubchandani, J., McKinney, M., & Braun, R. (2013). Racial/Ethnic Disparities in Chronic Diseases of Youths and Access to Health Care in the United States. BioMed Research International. Retrieved from https://www.ncbi.nlm.nih.gov/pmc/articles/PMC3794652/.

2. www.cdc.gov. (2017). Autism Spectrum Disorder, Data & Statistics. [online] Available at: https://www.cdc.gov/ncbddd/autism/data.html

3. www.cdc.gov. (2012). 10 Leading Causes of Death by Age Group, United States - 2012. [online] Retrieved from https://www.cdc.gov/injury/wisqars/pdf/leading_causes_of_death_by_age_group_2012-a.pdf.

4. Woolsey/Rosebud, G. (2012, September 13). GMO Inside | GMO Timeline: A History of Genetically Modified Foods. Retrieved from http://www.gmoinside.org/gmo-timeline-a-history-genetically-modified-foods/

5. Nachman, D., Hardy, D., Matter, C., Bhave, A., & Penn, S. (Producers). (2015). The Human Experiment [Motion picture]. United States: KTF Films.

6. Toxic Chemicals. (2017, April 06). Retrieved from https://www.nrdc.org/issues/toxic-chemicals

7. EWG.org (n.d.). Toxic babies. Retrieved from https://www.ewg.org/enviroblog/2009/04/toxic-babies#.Wpj62hPwZE4

Chapter 3 - Listen To Your Body - Whatever That Means... - by Ky-Lee Hanson

1. Canada, G. O. (2018, February 23). Food and other selected items, average retail prices (Prices). Retrieved from http://www.statcan.gc.ca/tables-tableaux/sum-som/l01/cst01/econ155a-eng.htm

2. Homeostasis. (2018, February 28). Retrieved from https://en.wikipedia.org/wiki/Homeostasis

3. Hauser, R. (2016, January 28). Soy-rich diet may offset BPA's effects on fertility. Retrieved from https://www.hsph.harvard.edu/news/hsph-in-the-news/soy-rich-diet-may-offset-bpas-effects-on-fertility/

4. Zhou, J.-R., Yu, L., Mai, Z., & Blackburn, G. L. (2004). COMBINED INHIBITION OF ESTROGEN-DEPENDENT HUMAN BREAST CARCINOMA BY SOY AND TEA BIOACTIVE COMPONENTS IN MICE. International Journal of Cancer. Journal International Du Cancer, 108(1), 8–14. http://doi.org/10.1002/ijc.11549

5. Publishing, H. H. (n.d.). Getting your vitamins and minerals through diet. Retrieved from https://www.health.harvard.edu/womens-health/getting-your-vitamins-and-minerals-through-diet

6. Dirt Poor: Have Fruits and Vegetables Become Less Nutritious? (n.d.). Retrieved from https://www.scientificamerican.com/article/soil-depletion-and-nutrition-loss/

7. The Journal of the American College of Nutrition. (2016, December 14). Retrieved from http://americancollegeofnutrition.org/content/the-journal

8. Kushi Institute. (n.d.). Retrieved from https://www.kushiinstitute.org/

9. Organics Consumers Association. (n.d.). Retrieved from https://www.organicconsumers.org/

Chapter 4 - Libertaing Choice: Mindful Eating - by Effie Mitskopoulos

1. Dispenza, J. (2012). Breaking the habit of being yourself. New York: Hay House Inc.

2. Vangsness, S. (2016, April 13). Mastering the mindful meal. Brigham Health. Retrieved from http://www.brighamandwomens.org/Patients_Visitors/pcs/nutrition/services/healtheweightfor-women/special_topics/intelihealth0405.aspx.

3. Kabat-Zinn, J. (1990). Full Catastrophe Living. New York: Delta Trade Paperbacks.

4. Davis, D., & Hayes, J.A. (2012). What are the benefits of mindfulness? American Psychological Association 43(7), 64. Retrieved from http://www.apa.org/monitor/2012/07-08/ce-corner.aspx

5. Healthline Editorial Team, medically reviewed by Butler, N. (2016, June 2,). Mood food: Can what you eat affect your happiness?Healthline. Retrieved from http://healthline.com/health/mood-food-can-what-you-eat-affect-your-happiness#overview1

6. Wallis D.J; Hetherington M.M. (2004). Stress and eating: the effects of ego-threat and cognitive demand on food intake in restrained and emotional eaters. Appetite. 43, 39-46.

7. Gibson, E. L. (2006). Emotional influences on food choice: Sensory, physiological and psychological pathways. Physiology & Behaviour. 89(1), 53-61.

8. MIT Medical. (2017). Eating healthfully. Retrieved from https://medical.mit.edu/community/eating-healthfully https://medical.mit.edu/sites/default/files/hunger-scale.pdf and https://medical.mit.edu/sites/default/files/mindful_eating_journal.pdf

9. Blass, E.M., Anderson, D. R., Kirkorian, H.L., Pempek, T.A., Price, I., & Koleini, M.F. (2006). On the road to obesity: Television viewing increases intake of high-density foods. Physiology & Behaviour. 88, 597-604

10. Van Der Wal, R.C., & Van Dillen, L.F. (2013). Leaving a flat taste in your mouth: Task load reduces taste perception. Psychological Science. 124, 1277-1284.

11. Division of Nutrition and Physical Activity. (2006, May). Do increased portion sizes affect how much we eat? Research to Practice Series No. 2. Atlanta: Centres for Disease Control and Prevention. Retrieved from https://www.cdc.gov/nccdphp/dnpa/nutrition/pdf/portion_size_research.pdf

12. CBC News. (2014, March 4). Canada's obesity rates triple in less than 30 years. Retrieved from www.cbc.ca/news/health/canada-s-obesity-rates-triple-in-less-than-30-years-1.2558365

13. Wansink, B., Painter, J.E., & North, J. (2005). Bottomless bowls: Why visual cues of portion size may influence intake. Obesity Research and Clinical Practice. 13, 93-100.

14. Diabetes Canada. (2017). Portion guide. Retrieved from http://www.diabetes.ca/diabetes-and-you/healthy-living-resources/diet-nutrition/portion-guide

15. Monroe, J.T. (2015). Mindful eating principles and practices. American Journal of LifestyleMedicine. 9(3):217-220.

Chapter 6 - Healthy Self = Heal "Thy Self - by Charleyne Oulton

1. Irish Twins. (n.d.). The Dictionary of American Slang. Retrieved from Dictionary.com website http://www.dictionary.com/browse/irish-twins

2. WebMD (n.d.). Stress Symptoms. Retrieved from https://www.webmd.com/balance/stress-management/stress-symptoms-effects_of-stress-on-the-body#2

3 Gunnars, Kris (2017, April,19). 11 proven health benefits of Quinoa. Healthline. Retrieved from http://www.healthline.com/nutrition/11-proven-benefits-of-quinoa#section1

Chapter 7 - Mindful Living For The Empowered Woman - by Kelly Spencer

1. Go AS, Mozaffarian D, Roger VL, Benjamin EJ, Berry JD, Borden WB, Bravata DM, Dai S, Ford ES, Fox CS, Franco S, Fullerton HJ, Gillespie C, Hailpern SM, Heit JA, Howard VJ, Huffman MD, Kissela BM, Kittner SJ, Lackland DT, Lichtman JH, Lisabeth LD, Magid D, Marcus GM, Marelli A, Matchar DB, McGuire DK, Mohler ER, Moy CS, Mussolino ME, Nichol G, Paynter NP, Schreiner PJ, Sorlie PD, Stein J, Turan TN, Virani SS, Wong ND, Woo D, Turner MB; on behalf of the American Heart Association Statistics Committee and Stroke Statistics Subcommittee. Heart disease and stroke statistics—2013 update: A report from the American Heart Association.Circulation. 2013;127:e6-e245.

2. Braden, G. (2004). the God Code. Carlsbad, CA: Hayhouse.

3. Emoto, D. M. (2004). The Hidden Messages in Water. Hillsboro: Beyond Words Publishing.

4. Tilman, P. O. (2015). Global diets link environmental sustainability and human health. University of Minnesota: Nature.

5. Suzuki, D. (2017, june 5th). Aquaculture Stewardship Council certified salmon isn't a "Good Alternative". Retrieved from David Suzuki Foundation: https://davidsuzuki.org/press/aquaculture-stewardship-council-certified-salmon-isnt-good-alternative/

6. Institute, M. C. (n.d.). Destructive Fishing. Retrieved from marine-conservation.org: https://marine-conservation.org/what-we-do/program-areas/how-we-fish/destructive-fishing/

7. Glass, E. (2013, august 2nd). The Environmental Impact of GMOs. Retrieved from One Green Planet: http://www.onegreenplanet.org/animalsandnature/the-environmental-impact-of-gmos/

Chapter 8 - High Intensity For The Intense Woman - by Ashly Hill

1. Perry, C. G., Heigenhauser, G. J., Bonen, A., & Spriet, L. L. (2008). High-intensity aerobic interval training increases fat and carbohydrate metabolic capacities in human skeletal muscle. Applied Physiology, Nutrition, and Metabolism, 33(6), 1112-1123.

2. Cameron-Smith, P. D. (2017, March 14). HIIT Benefits & Excess Post-Exercise Oxygen Consumption – Les Mills. Retrieved from https://www.lesmills.com/knowledge/fitness-research/feel-the-afterburn/

3. Gulati, M. (Ed.). (n.d.). Women's unique risk factors. Heart and Stroke Foundation Canada. Retrieved May 31, 2017, from http://www.heartandstroke.ca/heart/risk-and-prevention/womens-unique-risk-factors

4. What is Heart Disease? (n.d.). National Heart, Lung, and Blood Institute. Retrieved from https://www.nhlbi.nih.gov/health/educational/hearttruth/lower-risk/what-is-heart-disease.htm

5. Viola, V., Lina B., Roberto, C., Cor, D., W., Maria, D., Alistair, H., Akos, K. Mario, M., Axel, P., & Raffaele, B., (2011). Ischaemic heart disease in women: are there sex differences in pathophysiology and risk factors?: Position Paper from the Working Group on Coronary Pathophysiology and Microcirculation of the European Society of Cardiology. 90(1), 9-17. doi:10.1093/cvr/cvq394

6. Read, A. (n.d.). Use Active Rest to Build More Muscle. Breaking Muscle. Retrieved from https://breakingmuscle.com/fitness/use-active-rest-to-build-more-muscle

7. Kehler, A. K., & Heinrich, K. M. (2015). A selective review of prenatal exercise guidelines since the 1950s until present: Written for women, health care professionals, and female athletes. Women and Birth, 28(4), e93-e98.

8. Census Canada (2016). Census 2016: The growing age gap, gender ratios and other key takeaways. The Globe and Mail. Retrieved from https://beta.theglobeandmail.com/news/national/census-2016-statscan/article34882462/?ref=www.theglobeandmail.com&

9. Stöppler, MD, M. C. (n.d.). Menopause Age, Early Peri/Post Symptoms (Weight Gain) & Treatment. Retrieved from http://www.medicinenet.com/menopause/article.htm

10. Mendoza, N., De Teresa, C., Cano, A., Godoy, D., Hita-Contreras, F., Lapotka, M., ... & Rodríguez-Alcalá, L. (2016). Benefits of physical exercise in postmenopausal women. Maturitas, 93, 83-88.

11. Angelo.T, Tremblay, A., Simoneau, J. A., & Bouchard, C. (1994). Impact of exercise intensity on body fatness and skeletal muscle metabolism. Metabolism, 43(7), 814-818.

Chapter 9 - Fit Way Of Life - Deirdre Slattery

1. U.S National Library of Medicine. (2017, May 04). What are the treatment options for heavy periods? Retrieved from https://www.ncbi.nlm.nih.gov/pubmedhealth/PMH0072477/

2. Gottfried, S., MD. (n.d.). How To Overcome PMS and Painful Periods. Retrieved from http://www.saragottfriedmd.com/how-to-overcome-pms-and-painful-periods/

3. Chromium(III) picolinate. (2018, April 03). Retrieved from https://en.wikipedia.org/wiki/Chromium(III)_picolinate

4. Marks, L. (2016, May 09). Chromium Picolinate - Side Effects, Dosage, Interactions - Drugs. Retrieved from https://www.everydayhealth.com/drugs/chromium-picolinate

Chapter 10 - You Don't Get The Ass You Want By Sitting On It - Paula Man

1. Bernstein, L., Henderson, B., Hanisch, R., Sulliven-Halley, J.,Ross, R. (1994, Sept 21). "Physical exercise reduces the risk of breast cancer in Women under 40." J.N.C.I.- Journal of the National Cancer Institute

2. Kohrt, W.M, Landt. M, and Birge, S.J. Jr. (1996, Nov 1). Exercise reduces leptin levels. J.C.E.M. Journal of Clinical Endocrinology and Metabolism

3. Popova, M. (2016, July 08). How Long It Takes to Form a New Habit., Retrieved from https://www.brainpickings.org/2014/01/02/how-long-it-takes-to-form-a-new-habit/

Chapter 12 - Getting My Menstrual Cycle On Point - Amy Rempel

1. Babcock, J. (2017, December 04). Birth control pills before having kids? Your breast cancer risk jumps to 1-in-5. Retrieved from https://draxe.com/birth-control-pills/

2. Signs and Symptoms of Blood Clots. (n.d.). National Blood Clot Alliance. Retrieved March 02, 2018, from https://www.stoptheclot.org/learn_more/blood_clot_symptoms__dvt.htm

3. Publishing, H.H (n.d). Becoming A Vegetarian. Harvard Health Publishing. Retrieved March 02, 2018, from https://www.health.harvard.edu/staying-healthy/becoming-a-vegetarian

4. Total Wellness Publishing. (2017). The Essential Life 3rd Edition.

5. Greger, M., M.D. FALCM . (2016, September 13). Estrogen in Animal Products. Retrieved from https://nutritionfacts.org/2016/09/13/estrogen-animal-products/

6. Shahbazi,Yasser; Malekinejad, Hassan; Tajik, Hossein. (2011, April 26). Determination of naturally occurring estrogenic hormones in cow's and river buffalo's meat. PubMed. U.S National Library of Medicine. National Institute of Health. Retrieved from ,https://www.ncbi.nlm.nih.gov/pubmed/?term=estrogen+in+beef+and+river+buffalo%5C

7. Corio, Laura MD. (2011, October 11). F is for Fibroids [Web log post]. Retrieved from https://blogs.webmd.com/womens-health/2011/10/f-is-for-fibroids.html

8. Goldberg, Joseph. (2017, October 13). Depression and PMS. WebMD, https://www.webmd.com/women/pms/depression-pms

9. Wszelaki, Magdalena. How the Pill Can Seriously Affect a Woman's Health. Hormones & Balance, https://www.hormonesbalance.com/articles/pill-can-seriously-affect-womans-health/.

10. Living With: Premenstrual Dysphoric Disorder. Psych Guides, https://www.psychguides.com/guides/living-with-premenstrual-dysphoric-disorder/.

11 Emnett, Amy. Clary Sage Essential Oil. The School for Aromatic Studies, https://aromaticstudies.com/clary-sage-essential-oil/.

12 (Tiberian, Janet. "Foods That May Help Boost Your Estrogen and Testosterone Levels." MDVIP, https://www.mdvip.com/about-mdvip/blog/foods-to-boost-estrogen-testosterone-levels.

Chapter 13 - Empower and Heal Your Body, Mind, And Soul With Purpose, Passion, and Kindness - by Tania Jane Moraes Vaz

1. National Infertility Awareness Week. (n.d.). Retrieved from https://infertilityawareness.org/

2. Azziz, R., MD, MPH, & Ehrmann, D., MD (Eds.). (n.d.). Polycystic Ovary Syndrome (PCOS). Retrieved from https://www.hormone.org/diseases-and-conditions/womens-health/polycystic-ovary-syndrome

3. Watson, S., D. R. Wilson PhD, MSN, RN, IBCLC, AHN-BC, CHT, Ed.(2017, September 27). Polycystic Ovary Syndrome (PCOS): Symptoms, Causes, and Treatment. Retrieved from https://www.healthline.com/health/polycystic-ovary-disease?m=2#overview1

Chapter 14 - Allow Your Body To Heal From The Inside Out - Allison Marschean

1. Hebrews. (2011). In Holy Bible. Nashville, TN: Biblica.

2. G.K., Roper. (2012). Lupus Awareness Survey for the Lupus Foundation of America [Executive Summary Report]. Washington, D.C.

3. Rubin, R. L. (2005). Drug-induced lupus. Toxicology, 209(2), 135-147.

Chapter 15 - Acupuncture To My Rescue - Jenna Knight

1. Acupuncture. Gale Encyclopedia of Alternative Medicine. Retrieved from Encyclopedia.com: http://www.encyclopedia.com/medicine/encyclopedias-almanacs-transcripts-and-maps/acupuncture-1

2. MRI Reveals Acupuncture Modulates Brain Activity. (2015, April 07). Retrieved from www.healthcmi.com/Acupuncture-Continuing-Education-News/1449-mri-reveals-acupuncture-modulates-brain-activity

3. He, Tian, Wen Zhu, Si-Qi Du, Jing-Wen Yang, Fang Li, Bo-Feng Yang, Guang-Xia Shi, and Cun-Zhi Liu. "Neural mechanisms of acupuncture as revealed by fMRI studies." Autonomic Neuroscience (2015).

Chapter 17 - An Italian Lesson In Balance - Samantha Cifelli

1. Eating Well editors (2009). Eating well by color. Retrieved from http://www.eatingwell.com/food_news_origins/seasonal_local/eatingwell_in_season/eating_well_by_color.

2. Robyn Sirgley (2015). 6 hormone-balancing foods For women. Retrieved from https://www.mindbodygreen.com/0-20217/6-hormone-balancing-foods-for-women.html.

3. Maureen Callahan (2010). 7 healthy foods that deliver just what women need. Retrieved from http://www.cookinglight.com/eating-smart/nutrition-101/foods-for-women#best-foods-for-women.

4. Annie Daly (2014). 5 reasons to eat more avocados. Retrieved from http://www.womenshealthmag.com/food/eat-more-avocados. The top 10 arugula health benefits. Retrieved from http://superfood-profiles.com/arugula-health-benefits.

5. Megan Ware (2016). Peaches: health benefits, facts, research. Retrieved from http://www.medicalnewstoday.com/articles/274620.php.

Chapter 18 - Plants On Plates: Possibilities, Passion, A Path, And A Plan - Margie Cook

1. Endocrine Disruptors. (n.d.). Retrieved from https://www.niehs.nih.gov/health/topics/agents/endocrine/index.cfm

Beef Up Your Meal - The Unexpected Meal Topper Proteins - Ky-Lee Hanson

1. McClees, H. (2015, January 20). 5 Soy-Free Vegan Foods That Have More Protein Than Beef. Retrieved from http://www.onegreenplanet.org/natural-health/soy-free-vegan-foods-that-have-more-protein-than-beef/

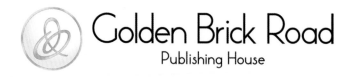

Golden Brick Road
Publishing House

Locking arms and helping each other down
their Golden Brick Road

At Golden Brick Road Publishing House, we lock arms with ambitious people and create success through a collaborative, supportive, and accountable environment. We are a boutique shop that caters to all stages of business around a book. We encourage women empowerment, and gender and cultural equality by publishing single author works from around the world, and creating in-house collaborative author projects for emerging and seasoned authors to join.

Our authors have a safe space to grow and diversify themselves within the genres of poetry, health, sociology, women's studies, business, and personal development. We help those who are natural born leaders, step out and shine! Even if they do not yet fully see it for themselves. We believe in empowering each individual who will then go and inspire an entire community. Our Director, Ky-Lee Hanson, calls this: The Inspiration Trickle Effect.

If you want to be a public figure that is focused on helping people and providing value, but you do not want to embark on the journey alone, then we are the community for you.

To inquire about our collaborative writing opportunities or to bring your own idea into vision, reach out to us at:

www.goldenbrickroad.pub